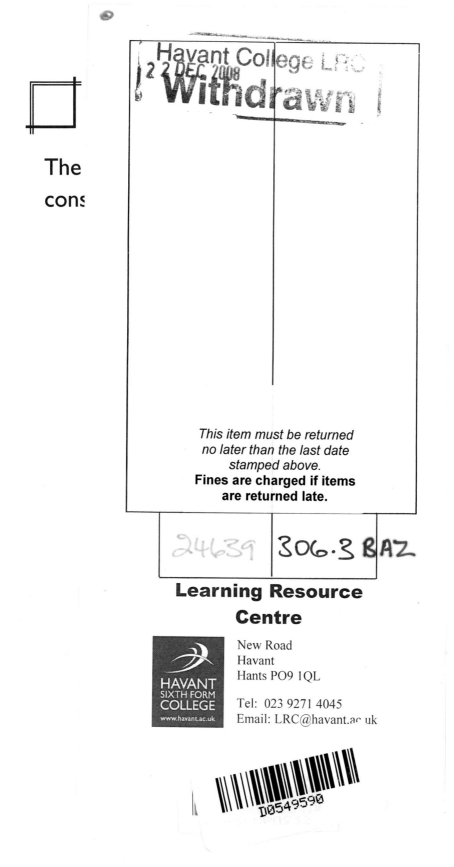

The

cons

Learning Resource Centre

Applying social psychology
Series editor: Stephen Sutton

Published and forthcoming titles

Richard P. Bagozzi, Zeynep Gürhan-Canli and Joseph R. Priester: *The Social Psychology of Consumer Behaviour*

Mark Conner and Christopher J. Armitage: *The Social Psychology of Food*

Steve Sussman and Susan L. Ames: *The Social Psychology of Drug Abuse*

The social psychology of
consumer behaviour

Richard P. Bagozzi, Zeynep Gürhan-Canli
and Joseph R. Priester

Open University Press
Buckingham · Philadelphia

Open University Press
Celtic Court
22 Ballmoor
Buckingham
MK18 1XW

email: enquiries@openup.co.uk
world wide web: www.openup.co.uk

and

325 Chestnut Street
Philadelphia, PA 19106, USA

First Published 2002

A catalogue record of this book is available from the British Library

ISBN   0 335 20722 7 (pb)   0 335 20723 5 (hb)

Library of Congress Cataloging-in-Publication Data
Bagozzi, Richard P.
    The social psychology of consumer behaviour / Richard P. Bagozzi,
Zeynep Gürhan-Canli, Joseph R. Priester.
        p. cm. – (Applying social psychology)
    Includes bibliographical references and index.
    ISBN 0-335-20723-5 – ISBN 0-335-20722-7 (pbk.)
    1. Consumption (Economics)–Social aspects. 2. Consumer behavior.
3. Consumers–Psychology. I. Gürhan-Canli, Zeynep, 1968–
II. Priester, Joseph R., 1960– III. Title. IV. Series.

HB801 .B267 2002
306.3–dc21   2001056007

Typeset by Graphicraft Limited, Hong Kong
Printed in Great Britain by St Edmundsbury Press Limited, Bury St Edmunds, Suffolk

Contents

Series editor's foreword

Social psychology is sometimes criticized for not being sufficiently 'relevant' to everyday life. The Applying Social Psychology series challenges this criticism. It is organized around applied topics rather than theoretical issues, and is designed to complement the highly successful Mapping Social Psychology series edited by Tony Manstead. Social psychologists, and others who take a social-psychological perspective, have conducted research on a wide range of interesting and important applied topics such as drug use, work, politics, the media, crime and environmental issues. Each book in the new series takes a different applied topic and reviews relevant social-psychological ideas and research. The books are texts rather than research monographs. They are pitched at final year undergraduate level, but will also be suitable for students on Masters level courses as well as researchers and practitioners working in the relevant fields. Although the series has an applied emphasis, theoretical issues are not neglected. Indeed, the series aims to demonstrate that theory-based applications of social psychology can contribute to our understanding of important applied topics.

The latest book in the series addresses consumer behaviour, defined broadly as the acquisition, use and disposal of products, services, ideas and practices. The book focuses on the 'why and how' of consumer behaviour: why people buy what they do and how they go about doing this. The authors are sophisticated theorists as well as empirical researchers. Their approach draws not only on social-psychological theories of attitude formation, attitude-behaviour relations, and attitude change but also on ideas from cognitive and emotional psychology. The reader will find lucid and detailed descriptions and critiques of leading theories such as the elaboration likelihood model of persuasion and the theory of planned behaviour. The authors also present their own theories of consumer action, the 'theory of trying' and the more recent model of goal-directed behaviour, which aims to integrate automatic, cognitive, emotional, and volitional factors to capture the complexity of determinants of consumer behaviour. The book is both an authoritative overview of what is known about consumer behaviour and a valuable source of interesting and novel ideas for future research.

Stephen Sutton

List of figures and tables

Figures

Tables

Acknowledgements

We are especially grateful to Janet Nightingale for all the work and support she gave us during this project. Janet not only entered the final manuscript, but also served as a copy-editor with regard to references and she indexed the book. She also cajoled us to keep on schedule. We are most appreciative of her input.

1

Introduction: overview of consumer behaviour

Consumer behaviour consists of the psychological and social processes people undergo in the acquisition, use and disposal of products (for example automobiles), services (for example professional laundry), ideas (for example spiritual beliefs) and practices (for example regular breast self-examinations). Sometimes consumer behaviour is studied from the point of view of a marketer, whereby focus is on a particular brand (for example Movado wristwatches) and how to get people to buy it. More often academic researchers study consumer behaviour from the point of view of applied or even basic behavioural and social sciences. Emphasis here is on understanding and explaining why people buy what they do and how (intrapersonally and socially) they go about doing this.

The why and how of consumer behaviour have been approached in many ways and by multiple methods. Consumer researchers with an anthropological or sociological bent have studied consumption as an integral part of culture and social relationships. Their methodology has been largely qualitative consisting of participant observation, case studies, and the application of various ethnomethodological practices. Occasionally surveys have been employed by these researchers. Clinical and classically trained psychologists were early shapers of the field of consumer behaviour and did much to codify underlying motivations of consumers, as well as apply principles of learning, **perception** and personality to consumer research. Typically, psychologists used depth interviews or focus groups, but sometimes experiments and surveys as well. The field currently sees a flowering of interpretative research by researchers trained in anthropology, psychology and sociology.

Since the late 1970s, the core of consumer research has been located in inquiry performed from the point of view of social psychology and cognitive psychology, with recent insights provided by behavioural decision researchers as well. Information processing drives this research, and the experimental method, and to a lesser extent survey research, is the preferred approach.

This book presents research into consumer behaviour from the point of view of social psychology. Unlike other applied areas of psychology which arose from and continue to be influenced primarily by psychologists, the social psychology of consumer behaviour owes its modern form and content to the influence of an eclectic group of researchers and practitioners from marketing and all the social and behavioural sciences, as well as many subfields within psychology. At the same time, the study of the social psychology of consumer behaviour has been shaped profoundly by the Association for Consumer Research (ACR, founded in 1970) and the *Journal of Consumer Research* (*JCR*), an interdisciplinary scholarly publication begun in 1974. The latter has been joined in recent years by the *Journal of Consumer Psychology*.

The mix of traditions and perspectives in consumer research makes for an amorphous body of knowledge and a challenge of what to include and what to exclude from our presentation. We erred on the side of inclusion by introducing research from cognitive psychology and emotional psychology as they inform or directly interface with contemporary social psychology in consumer behaviour. Primarily because of space limitations, and given their somewhat more distant relationship to social psychology, we explicitly omitted discussion of many contributions from anthropology, behavioural decision theory, behaviourism (see Foxall 1996, 1997), economics, political science and sociology.

We strove to present ideas and research to aid thinking. The focus is on fundamental principles as grounded in basic research, rather than on facts to be remembered. For excellent compendiums of knowledge about consumer behaviour in its broadest senses, the reader is referred to Wilkie (1994) and Engel et al. (1995). East (1997), Kardes (1999) and Hoyer and MacInnis (2001) provide fine coverage of the science and practice of consumer behaviour.

Although the research presented herein was generated largely by scholars in the western tradition, it would be a mistake to conclude that the point of view is limited to ideas situated strictly in that tradition. Today leading researchers hail from all over the world and have brought their unique perspectives to bear on the subject matter. To be sure, there are strong biases in the development of the field and in the current tastes of editors, reviewers and other gatekeepers. But many of these barriers are under siege, and we see a flowering of debate and healthy and exciting ferment in contemporary research.

The cognitive paradigm held sway from the earliest days of the ACR and *JCR*. It continues its hegemony to this day. Nevertheless, we see a budding concern for the implications of cognition, as it applies to consumer behaviour writ large. To this end, the topics treated in this book begin with the foundation laid in attitude research, **emotion** and emerging explanations of consumer **action**, then scrutinize the effects of persuasive communication, and end with a comprehensive review of cognitive processes, which historically has been the heart of the field.

We hope that you will be motivated to study further the social psychology of consumer behaviour, after reading this book. We are confident that you will find the subject matter intriguing and more intricate than you might have thought, before considering the research detailed herein. We anticipate, too, that you will gain a better understanding of why and how you and others around you consume what you do.

The rest of the book is structured as follows. In Chapter 2, we introduce the idea of **attitudes**. Unidimensional conceptualizations of attitudes (especially the **expectancy-value model**) are considered, along with classic theoretical and measurement issues. Included in the discussion are treatments of the bases for attitudes as represented in **means-end chain theory** and **goals**. The presentation on attitudes concludes with new developments in multidimensional conceptualizations.

Chapter 3 reviews research into the emotional foundations of consumer behaviour, where **appraisal theories** and **circumplex models** are highlighted. This is followed by a discussion of key measurement issues in emotions. Next, the related topic of arousal is considered. Emotions are then viewed functionally as markers, mediators and moderators in consumer research. Finally, the chapter closes with presentations of the role of emotions in cognitive processing, customer **satisfaction** and social aspects of consumption.

Perhaps the most neglected area in consumer research is on consumer actions and how actions relate to attitudes, cognitive processes and emotion. Chapter 4 addresses these concerns by describing and critiquing three leading theories of action and introducing three surfacing alternatives. We then integrate many of the ideas in emergent research and end with a comprehensive framework for studying consumer action.

Chapter 5 looks into attitude change, particularly from the point of view of the elaboration likelihood model of **persuasion**. After a brief history of the evolution of learning theory, balance theory and the cognitive response movement, which provides an introduction and background to both persuasion models and the review of cognitive processes to be covered in Chapter 6, the basic principles of the elaboration likelihood model are covered. The chapter closes with brief considerations of the consequences of **elaboration**.

Cognitive processes are treated in Chapter 6. This is probably the single most researched area in the field and continues to spawn much inquiry. The specific topics covered are attention, perception, categorization, **schemas**, memory and inferences and information search. We might think of attitudes, emotion and cognitive processes as providing the basis or reasons for consumer action.

2

Attitudes: content, structure, processes

The study of attitudes has a long history in the field of consumer behaviour and an even longer history in social psychology. As far back as 1935, a leading psychologist noted: 'the concept of attitude is probably the most distinctive and indispensable concept in . . . social psychology' (Allport 1935: 198). It still is today.

What is an attitude?

The concept of attitude has an interesting history (Fleming 1967). Originally, the word attitude seems to have been used to signify a posture or inclination of one's body, so as to suggest a mental state or imply an action. This usage had its origins in French and Spanish from the Italian, *attitudine*, and the late Latin, *aptitudo* (*New Shorter Oxford English Dictionary*). In Italian, *attitudine* means aptitude (*Collins English–Italian, Italian–English Dictionary*). Today, most people in everyday discourse tend to use the word attitude to signify a state of mind in the sense of 'settled behaviour, as representing feeling or opinion' (*New Shorter Oxford English Dictionary*). Likewise, in Italian, attitude is now commonly translated, not as *attitudine*, but as *atteggiamento*, which means a point of view or mode of thinking (*Collins English–Italian, Italian–English Dictionary*).

In contrast to common usage, the meaning of attitude has undergone a technical evolution in social psychology and in applied fields. The most widely accepted definition of attitude conceives of it as an **evaluation**. Here are some examples:

Attitudes are . . . individuals' evaluations of objects.

(Gold with Douvan 1997: 65)

Attitude is a psychological tendency that is expressed by evaluating a particular entity with some degree of favor or disfavor.

(Eagly and Chaiken 1993: 1)

An attitude is an association in memory between an attitude object and an evaluation.

(Fazio 1989)

Eagly and Chaiken (1993: 1) note further that 'evaluating' 'refers to all classes of evaluative responding, whether overt or covert, cognitive, affective, or behavioral'. By 'evaluative', we generally mean expressing a judgement as to the value of something (*New Shorter Oxford English Dictionary*). Judgements are typically represented as good–bad, favourable–unfavourable, and so on.

The term attitude is a generic one and loosely subsumes other technical terms used in social psychology. When we have attitudes toward friends or respected others, we mean liking, attraction or even love. When we speak of people's attitudes toward subcategories of people, we mean prejudices, partiality or favouritism. Attitudes toward the self are called self-worth, self-esteem or self-image. Attitudes towards products, political candidates or services are sometimes termed preferences. Attitudes toward issues or ideas are designated opinions. Attitudes of employees toward work are known as job satisfaction. When people make inferences about their own attitudes we call these self-perceptions, about other people's attitudes, attributions. Even **values**, goals and motives might be considered sub-species of attitudes, as they refer to abstract end-states evaluated favourably or unfavourably. In sum, we have attitudes toward people ('I like Tony Blair'), ideas ('I am against capital punishment'), objects ('Double Diamond beer is my favourite'), places ('a holiday in the Caribbean appeals to me') and even ourselves ('I am basically a good person').

The one-dimensional model of attitude

A popular and influential conceptualization of attitude sees it as an indication of a person's position toward an issue or object along an evaluative continuum (for example Thurstone 1928; Fishbein 1967a; Petty and Cacioppo 1981, 1986). Attitude from this point of view is a singular, unidimensional evaluative response. A nice way to see this is to consider two ways that attitudes are frequently measured, in Figure 2.1: by Likert and **semantic differential** scaling techniques (Likert 1932; Osgood et al. 1957). The Likert items ask respondents to indicate their degree of agreement or disagreement, or whether they are neutral, on a 5-point scale. Of course, the continuum can be expanded to 7-point, 9-point or more graduated scales. The semantic differential items also capture a person's attitude as a matter of degree along an evaluative continuum and do so by use of bipolar adjectives. We have shown favourable–unfavourable and good–bad as examples, but others may include such instances as wise–foolish, punishing–rewarding, beautiful–ugly and useful–useless, depending on the attitudinal target and the researcher's purposes. Note, too, that we typically use a number of Likert or semantic

(a) *Likert scaling*: degree of support for the manner of electing presidents in the United States

1 The Electoral College should be eliminated.

+2	+1	0	−1	−2
Strongly agree	Agree	Neither agree nor disagree	Disagree	Strongly disagree

2 The president and vice president should be chosen on the basis of direct vote of the people.

1	2	3	4	5
Strongly agree	Agree	Neither agree nor disagree	Disagree	Strongly disagree

(b) *Semantic differential*

My attitude toward the Electoral College can be best described as:

favourable _____ ___ _____ _____ _____ ___ _____ unfavourable

extremely quite slightly neither slightly quite extremely

Bad _____ ___ _____ _____ _____ ___ _____ Good

−3   −2   −1   0   +1   +2   +3

Figure 2.1 Examples of items used to measure attitude along an evaluative continuum

differential items to measure a person's attitude in order to increase the reliability of measurement. But under the unidimensional conceptualization of attitude, each item is assumed to measure the same attitude.

Representation of unidimentional attitudes: the expectancy-value model

We often associate what a person believes and how important these **beliefs** are to them with their attitude. Imagine that a researcher wishes to discover the attitudes of consumers toward a particular restaurant and to understand more fully the basis for, or senses of, the expressed attitudes. We might expect people's favourability or unfavourability toward the restaurant to vary as a global evaluation, as well as in particular judgements and evaluations of such restaurant attributes as quality of food and service, convenience of location and hours of operation, aesthetic ambience and parking facilities. One way to capture consumers' attitudes toward the restaurant (A_{res}) is by use of the following equation, which is a specific instance of the 'expectancy-value model' of attitude:

$$A_{res} = b_{fq}e_{fq} + b_{sq}e_{sq} + b_{lc}e_{lc} + b_{ho}e_{ho} + b_{aa}e_{aa} + b_{pf}e_{pf} \qquad (2.1)$$

where A_{res} refers to a consumer's overall attitude toward (that is, evaluation of) the restaurant, the b_i's are beliefs or judgements about the characteristics of the restaurant (for example b_{lc} is the consumer's belief about the location convenience of the restaurant, which might be measured, say, on a 5-point scale going from 'not at all convenient' to 'very convenient'), the e_i's capture the consumer's evaluations or possibly importances of the characteristics of the restaurant (for example e_{lc} is the consumer's evaluation of location convenience, which might be measured on a 5-point scale going from 'not at all important to me' to 'very important to me') and fq = food quality, sq = service quality, ho = hours of operation, aa = aesthetic ambience and pf = parking facilities. In words, equation 2.1 says, one's global attitude toward the restaurant equals or is a function of the sum of the products of one's beliefs that the restaurant possesses certain attributes and one's appraisal of how important (or good–bad) those attributes are for the consumer.

The expectancy-value attitude model is expressed in general form as follows:

$$A_{obj} = \sum_{i=1}^{n} b_i e_i \qquad (2.2)$$

where A_{obj} is one's attitude toward an object (for example product, service, person, place, idea), b_i and e_i are beliefs and evaluations, respectively, about attributes of the attitudinal object, and the multiplicative products of beliefs and evaluations are summed over n attributes. The origins of the expectancy-value model go back to ancient philosophers, particularly Aristotle. More recently, the model owes its form and content to early work by psychologists Edwards (1954), in his formulation of 'subjective expected utility theory', and Peak (1955), in his development of motivational content in attitude theory. Detailed developments and reviews of research on expectancy-value models can be found in Fishbein and Ajzen (1975) and Ajzen and Fishbein (1980). See also Feather (1982) and Dabholkar (1999). In addition to objects, attitudes can be expressed toward actions (A_{act}). For now, we limit focus to A_{obj} as opposed to A_{act}.

It is not an exaggeration to claim that the expectancy-value model is the most widely applied representation of attitude across many disciplines. One reason for this is that the expectancy-value model encapsulates two basic determinants of decision making: namely, our beliefs and our evaluations about attributes of an object of potential value to us. These determinants reflect, respectively, rational or reasoned aspects of our behaviour, as well as motivational. Another reason is the simplicity of the model. All things equal, scientists and practitioners prefer simple over complex formulations as a matter of aesthetics, if not values favouring parsimony.

Another reason behind the appeal of the expectancy-value model is the policy implications it suggests. The deceptively simple model offers multiple ways by which a change agent (for example marketer, health provider, political consultant) can attempt to influence and control the behaviours of others. Wilkie (1994) describes five strategies for attitude change: change consumer beliefs about one's own attributes, add new attributes, increase the importance of existing attributes, decrease the importance of weak attributes, and change beliefs about competitors' attributes. Attitude change is an important managerial objective and finds currency in the strategic tool known as brand positioning (for example Shocker and Srinivasan 1979; Green and Krieger 1992; Griffen and Hauser 1993) and in consumer choice models (for example Gensch and Svestka 1984; Green and Srinivasan 1990; Meyer and Kahn 1991; P.E. Green et al. 1993).

The managerial uses of the expectancy-value model rest on its validity as a representation of attitude formation and change. For a classic explication of the theory behind attitude formation and change in this regard, as well as empirical support, see Lutz (1975, 1977). Interesting commentary on the distinction between attitude formation and change can be found in the Carnegie-Mellon University Marketing Seminar (1978) and Lutz (1978). See also Bagozzi (1982: 570–4) and Bettman et al. (1975).

Unresolved issues with the expectancy-value model

Determination of beliefs

Many questions remain unanswered about expectancy-value models. An important issue is how to identify the beliefs that enter the model in equation 2.2. Our objective should be to identify those beliefs that actually constitute or determine one's global attitude. But to establish this in as definitive a way as possible, we must rely on evidence of some sort. The evidence might be observational and logical. For example, we might ask one person what their beliefs are about a new computer. How useful are its features? Is it easy to use? The consumer can assess how useful and easy to use the computer is as a matter of degree. These make up the consumer's beliefs. But how do we know that they relate to the consumer's attitude toward the new computer? One way to ascertain this is to ask the consumer to express their attitude and beliefs at different points in time and observe how strongly they correspond across time. Does a very favourable attitude at time 1 correspond to high scores on usefulness and ease of use at that point in time? Or if the attitude is less favourable at a future point in time, do the beliefs match analogously?

Alternatively, to ascertain the relationship between a consumer's attitude and beliefs, we might present different levels of attributes of a computer in different combinations, or present different computers, and ask the consumer to provide their attitudes and beliefs for each combination or each computer. Again, the correspondence between attitudes and beliefs should be consistent, if we are to conclude that attitudes and beliefs are related.

The above discussion focused on one consumer, and we discussed the varying of time, attributes or objects (that is, computers) to achieve enough deviations to perform a logical comparison between levels of beliefs about attributes and levels of overall attitude. These 'within-subjects' analyses can be made formal and put to statistical tests so as to quantitatively estimate the degree of correlation between beliefs and attitudes. More common is to achieve variability by performing 'across-subjects' analyses where a sample of consumers is asked to express attitudes and beliefs with respect to a new computer, say. Then if those consumers who judge that the computer scores low, medium or high on salient attributes also score low, medium or high, respectively, on their global attitudes, we may infer that we have identified beliefs that relate to attitudes for the people under study. Here, too, special statistical procedures can be used to establish this quantitatively.

But a number of problems should be pointed out. Can we assume that the observation of statistically significant correlations between beliefs and attitudes, as determined above, confirms the expectancy-value model? No, not necessarily. Remember that it is the multiplicative product between beliefs and evaluations that are hypothesized to form or produce one's attitude, under the expectancy-value model, and not merely one's beliefs in isolation. I may believe that the new IBM computer is exceedingly fast in performing computations, but this belief may be unrelated with my attitude because speed of computation is not important to me (a computer may be used by me primarily as a word processor, for example). Someone else needing a computer to do sophisticated mathematical analyses may require high speed computations, and therefore, we may find that belief of high speed and a favourable attitude are positively related for this person.

Because statistical analyses require variability, we need to select beliefs for a sample of people (in the case of between subjects designs) or for a sample of objects or across points in time (for within subjects designs). Statistical issues that we will not consider here are the implications of the assumed homogeneity in correlation coefficients across people (presumed in the former design) and homogeneity in coefficients across objects or time (presumed in the latter design). The issue we wish to discuss now is how to select beliefs for a sample of people (an analogous issue concerns the selection of beliefs across objects and time for within subjects analyses).

Ajzen and Fishbein (1980: 68 and Appendix A; see also Fishbein and Ajzen 1975: 218–22) developed a procedure for selecting **modal salient beliefs**, which are the set of beliefs that are notable and relevant in a given population. The procedure is as follows. A sample of people from a larger population that

Table 2.1   Modal salient beliefs for a sample of consumers appraising the Ford Escape XLS light-duty sports utility vehicle

Belief groupings	The Ford Escape XLS . . .	Frequency of mentions
1	manoeuvres nimbly	5
	feels 'sporty' when I drive it	13
	handles well	22
	is sure-footed on the road	6
2	soaks-up bumps	7
	is unphased by pot-holes	8
	gives a smooth ride	15
3	is a little heavy	9
	is under powered	17
	is sluggish on acceleration on freeways	24
	is a dog when towing my (trailer, boat, etc.)	7
4	lets me see the road well in front	27
	has plenty of glass	19
	lets me see cars to the rear and side well	12
5	is not cramped inside	16
	fits four adults plus luggage	17
	provides plenty of room	11
6	squeezes into small parking spaces	18
	is easy to drive in city traffic	15
	fits narrow streets	29
7	has beautiful upholstery	4
	has an elegant interior	11
	has a quality audio system	20
	has a really attractive exterior	6
8	is easy to get into and out of	35
	has convenient maintenance features	3
	has an easy to use tail-gate	22
	contains many neat features (for example glass holders)	8
9	is pretty good on gas	2
	has an extended warranty	5
	should be reliable	12
	is priced well	14

we wish to study is selected, and people are asked to list the advantages they believe an attitudinal object offers, then its disadvantages, and finally anything else associated with the object in their minds. Use of this three-step procedure might yield the modal salient beliefs listed in Table 2.1, which shows the beliefs that a sample of consumers might express about the Ford Escape, a new light-duty sports utility vehicle. Notice that we have grouped the beliefs into nine categories, where the wording for beliefs is expressed in people's own words. Ideally, we would like the beliefs within a group to be maximally similar, those between groups to be maximally different. Obviously, **categorization** according to similarity/difference is a subjective task and perhaps more a measure of the art and skill of a researcher than a precise science. But as a start, the categorization of beliefs seems to make sense. For example, 'under powered', 'sluggish on acceleration' and 'a dog when towing' appear to share a common meaning and reflect more or less synonyms for the same idea: namely, 'lacking in horsepower'. A number of subjective decisions are required when categorizing beliefs, but we will have no more to say about this in this monograph.

Once a set of beliefs has been generated and categorized, the next step is to select a subset for inclusion in a questionnaire to operationalize the expectancy-value model. Table 2.1 shows 32 distinct beliefs. An actual application of Ajzen and Fishbein's **belief elicitation** procedure would probably generate even more than 32 beliefs, depending on the attitudinal object and the size of, and knowledge of the people in, the sample. But even 32 beliefs would be unwieldy to include in most questionnaires, because of the need also to contain 32 corresponding evaluation items, as well as items for other variables. Moreover, it is unlikely that consumers really consider 32 distinct beliefs when evaluating an additudinal object. As a result, the number of beliefs for consideration must be pared. How is this to be done? We would like the number of beliefs chosen to represent the beliefs most important in attitude formation. But people differ in which beliefs are important in their individual decision making. Although the 32 beliefs uncovered above may be roughly representative of the major beliefs for the sample as a whole, most individual respondents would probably find only a subset relevant. In practice, researchers choose a manageable subset that covers as many respondents to be surveyed as possible. Depending on the attitudinal object and the familiarity of the target population of individuals with the object, it turns out that about 5 to 7 beliefs is sufficient in most cases, with as many as 10 to 12 needed on occasion. Here, of course, by number of beliefs, we are speaking about the categories generated through the above mentioned procedure.

Various rules of thumb have been used to select the actual number from the list of categories generated. To take an example, consider Table 2.2, which presents the categories shown in Table 2.1, but with summary labels, plus a few other categories. If one has reason to accept many beliefs, say 12, then the first 12 in Table 2.2 could be selected for inclusion in a subsequent study of attitudes. A frequently employed rule is to select all beliefs above a certain cut-off percentage. For complex and well-known attitudinal objects where people have many beliefs, one might select a low percentage cut-off: 20 per cent, for example. For a new attitudinal object, where a few or moderate amount of beliefs exist, a higher percentage might be chosen: say, 50 per cent. By the latter rule, we see that the top 5 beliefs in Table 2.2 would be chosen. Still another rule is to select a percentage of all beliefs elicited:

Table 2.2   Selection of modal salient beliefs for the Ford Escape XLS

Number designation	Summary labels for beliefs concerning the Ford Escape XLS	Frequency of mentions
1*	'Convenience' or 'functionality'	68
2	'Makes me feel powerful'	63
3*	'Sporty handling'	62
4*	'Under powered'	58
5*	'Good field of vision while driving'	57
6*	'Roomy'	46
7	'Makes me feel safe and secure'	45
8*	'Ease of driving and parking'	44
9*	'Aesthetic appeal'	41
10*	'Economical/reliable'	33
11*	'Smooth ride'	30
12	'Fun'	25
13	'Prestigious'	24
		Total 596

* Mentioned in Table 2.1

say, 75 per cent. By this criterion, we would designate the first 9 beliefs for inclusion in a questionnaire. Some argument can be made for selecting between 5 and 9 beliefs, based on the conclusion that people can hold, on average, only about 7 ± 2 pieces of information in working memory when weighing evidence during decision making (Fishbein and Ajzen 1975: 218).

The Ajzen and Fishbein (1980) belief elicitation procedure appears to introduce some arbitrariness into the selection of beliefs. The danger is that some salient beliefs are excluded, some extraneous beliefs included. A study by van der Plight and Eiser (1984) showed that non-salient beliefs correlate lower with attitudes than salient beliefs and do not contribute much to the prediction of attitudes over and above salient beliefs. Of course, it is important to remember that it is the sum of the products of beliefs times evaluations that is related to attitudes, under the expectancy-value model, and this may differ from the association between beliefs and attitudes, per se.

One approach to selecting beliefs that underlie people's evaluations of attitudinal objects is to provide people in a study with a list of beliefs and have them select those that they feel are the most salient (Budd 1986). This has the advantage of yielding salient beliefs that are idiosyncratic to each respondent (success here depends of course on the representativeness of the presented list). The disadvantage, when done in an across-subjects design, is that the coefficients relating belief-evaluation products to attitudes apply to a heterogeneous set of beliefs, and it is not possible therefore to make conclusions concerning which particular beliefs are salient for the sample at hand. Still another procedure is to permit respondents to generate their own beliefs (for example Towriss 1984; Rutter and Bunce 1989; Haddock and Zanna 1998). This produces an even better representation of salient beliefs than the aforementioned procedures, but shares the drawback with inferences drawn from procedures based on heterogeneous beliefs across respondents. A final alternative is to conduct within-subjects designs, as described above. This is fine as long as the assumptions of (a) homogeneity of coefficients across time or stimuli is met, as well as (b) non-autocorrelation of error terms and homogeneity of error variances. Davidson and Morrison (1983) provide some comparisons of the implications of using within-subjects versus across-subjects designs, but do not fully investigate the underlying statistical assumptions, especially for the within-subjects case. In sum, the issue of valid belief selection is an unresolved issue, and all approaches described in the literature to date offer trade-offs.

Interpretation of the relationship between expectancy-value products and attitudes

You may have noticed that, when referring to the relationship implied by the equality sign in equation 2.2, we have used a disjunction of words: for example, 'equals or is a function of', 'constitutes or determines' or 'forms or produces'. This was done deliberately to postpone discussion of the meaning of the equality sign.

The relationship between A_{obj} and Σbe can be interpreted in one or more of six senses (Bagozzi 1996). Again, until we introduce A_{act} below, we will speak of A_{obj}. But the comments here apply equally to A_{act}. Perhaps the earliest point of view was due to Fishbein (1967b) who claimed that A_{obj} and Σbe are related through identity: namely, A_{obj} is *defined* as the Σbe. Later, Fishbein and Ajzen (1975) took the point of view that the Σbe *determine* A_{obj}. That is, one's attitude is dependent on one's beliefs weighted by one's evaluations of the beliefs. The sequence of effects implied by this relationship is the most common interpretation of $A_{obj} = \Sigma be$. Indeed, the five strategies for attitude change discussed above assumed that $\Sigma be \rightarrow A_{obj}$. This perspective presumes that, by changing beliefs and/or evaluations, we can influence attitudes. Ajzen and Fishbein (1980: 72) reiterated this rendering of $A_{obj} = \Sigma be$ in their influential book: 'By measuring belief strength and evaluations . . . we can not only *predict* a given individual's attitude but we also obtain information about the *determinants* of his attitude'. Despite the intuitive appeal of such a diagnosis, Fishbein (1980) has shown a certain ambivalence toward the meaning of the equality sign in equation 2.2 and reverted back to a definitional interpretation:

if [we] were able to tap and accurately measure all of a person's salient behavioural beliefs and outcome evaluations, the indirect measure of attitude based on these beliefs and outcome evaluations summation (Σbe) should be perfectly correlated with a direct valid measure of attitude

(A_o). Thus the direct (A_o) and indirect measure (Σbe) would be interchangeable.

(Fishbein 1980: 84)

If they were interchangeable, then researchers would find the A_o representation most useful in research, for it requires fewer items than the Σbe to operationalize attitude. Perhaps the logic espoused by Fishbein (1980) and parsimony account for why A_o has been used more frequently than the Σbe. Nevertheless, Bagozzi (1981a, 1981b, 1982) showed that, even after correcting for measurement error, A_o and Σbe are distinct constructs and function differentially as predictors.

Given that A_{obj} and the Σbe are distinct constructs, what other possibilities might we use to interpret the relationship between the two? An unattractive alternative is that A_{obj} and the Σbe do not relate causally to each other but are correlated because they have common causes. A special case of this way of seeing the relationship is the viewpoint claiming that the constructs are *epiphenomena*. **Epiphenomenalism** is the philosophical doctrine that maintains that mental events (for example beliefs, attitudes, **intentions**) are caused by physical events in the brain but do not cause each other or anything else for that matter (for example McLaughlin 1989). Epiphenomenalism concerns issues of metaphysics and ontology and cannot be dismissed summarily. Nevertheless, we take the viewpoint in this monograph that mental events can be both caused by and cause physical events. Our approach is consistent with functionalism, monism and non-Cartesian forms of dualism. These topics are beyond the scope for discussion herein.

A fourth possibility is that A_{obj} and the Σbe are simply *unrelated*. Although this may be true on occasion empirically, we believe that the theories linking A_{obj} and the Σbe are compelling, and the wealth of empirical evidence argues against the interpretation of unrelatedness.

That the Σbe may be dependent on A_{obj} is a fifth reading of the relationship between the two. This is not as farfetched as it may seem. Researchers term this the **halo effect**, and some research supports this interpretation (for example Bagozzi 1996). The halo effect is defined as the influence of one's attitude on beliefs (and the product of beliefs times evaluations). Nisbett and Wilson (1977: 250) found, for example, that 'global evaluations of a person can induce altered evaluations of the person's attributes'. Likewise, Bagozzi (1996) found that attitudes toward giving blood affected beliefs about the consequences of giving blood and not vice versa.

The sixth possibility for a relationship between A_{obj} and the Σbe is one of **simultaneity**. Here A_{obj} and the Σbe influence each other reciprocally. This might occur over time as feedback effects, or nearly instantaneously as reciprocal causation. Not much research has been done investigating simultaneity. Simultaneity in the cross-section is difficult to defend conceptually, if one adheres to temporal priority from cause to effect as a criterion for causality (Bagozzi 1994a: 374–7). Longitudinally, it is possible for the Σbe at time 1 to affect A_{obj} at time 2, and A_{obj} at time 1 to affect Σbe at time 2. These 'cross-lagged' effects also have not been studied very often.

Thus, many possibilities underlie the seemingly simple relationship between A_{obj} and the Σbe implied by equation 2.1. Rather than seeing one of the six possibilities sketched about as necessarily being the definitive interpretation, we believe it is wise at this time to keep an open mind and acknowledge that any one of the following four relationships can happen in different circumstances: $\Sigma be \rightarrow A_{obj}$, $A_{obj} \rightarrow \Sigma be$, $\Sigma be \rightleftarrows A_{obj}$, and $\Sigma be \leftarrow (\text{common cause}) \rightarrow A_{obj}$, where the 'simultaneity' relation, $\rightleftarrows$, can occur instantaneously or over time and 'common cause' refers to one or more antecedents accounting for the covariation between Σbe and A_{obj}. In future research, we should ask under what conditions can the relationship be any one of the possibilities mentioned above. For example, Bagozzi (1996) found that the halo effect in a study of attitudes toward giving blood could be produced for positive beliefs and reduced for negative beliefs, when high physiological arousal is induced (see also Bagozzi 1994b). Much more research is needed into ascertaining the conditions governing the relationship between the Σbe and A_{obj}. Until we learn more about the myriad of factors likely to influence the relationship, it would be wise not to automatically presume any one particular relationship in any given situation. It is especially critical to gain more knowledge about the conditions behind the relationship because so much basic and applied research rests on the assumption of one sequence: namely, $\Sigma be \rightarrow A_{obj}$.

The evaluative component in the Σbe

Another unresolved issue under the expectancy-value model is how to interpret the second term in the Σbe, e. In the standard case, the $e_i s$ are taken to represent a person's evaluations, where evaluations mean assessments or appraisals of the goodness or badness of an attribute of an attitudinal object. Consistent with this interpretation, Ajzen and Fishbein (1980) advocated the use of good–bad semantic differential items to measure evaluations, and such items are indeed the most frequently used in practice. Based on research by Osgood et al. (1957), other measures of evaluation have been used as well, as redundant indicators of evaluations. For example, good–bad, advantageous–disadvantageous, nice–awful, wise–foolish, rewarding–punishing, safe–unsafe, valuable–worthless, clean–dirty, effective–ineffective and useful–useless are common adjective pairs used to measure evaluations.

Researchers, however, have not limited the measurement of attitudes to evaluations, per se, but have used in their place, or in addition, such measures of **affect** as pleasant–unpleasant, happy–sad, excited–depressed, satisfied–dissatisfied, like–dislike, pleased–angry, proud–ashamed, attractive–unattractive, joyful–joyless and enjoyable–unenjoyable. The problem with the above practices is that we risk confounding evaluations with affect. To compound the issue, researchers have not kept clear or distinct the theoretical meaning of evaluations and affect. Eagly and Chaiken (1993: 12) point out that Fishbein and Ajzen (1975) and many social psychologists have 'regarded affect as isomorphic with evaluation itself and used the terms interchangeably'. Yet, they maintain that '[e]valuation is the core of the attitude concept . . . and should not be equated with its less abstract manifestations in terms of particular beliefs, affects, behavior' (Eagly and Chaiken 1993: 666). We shall return to the above distinction later when we introduce the topic of multidimensional attitudes.

Still another confusion in the conceptualization and measurement of evaluations has been the replacement of evaluation in the expectancy-value model with importance weights, measured, say, by important–unimportant items (for example Wilkie 1994: 288). In fact, some consumer researchers have replaced beliefs and evaluations with measures of how satisfied–dissatisfied consumers are with each attribute of a product or service (or how satisfactory–unsatisfactory the consumer feels the attributes are) multiplied by how important–unimportant each attribute is for the consumer. For an early debate in the literature in this regard, see Cohen et al. (1972), Sheth (1972), Sheth and Talarzyk (1972), Wilkie and Pessemier (1973) and Mazis et al. (1975). The problem with the latter rendition of the expectancy-value model is that attribute satisfaction seems to confound beliefs and evaluations, and the addition of importance introduces yet another complication (Fishbein and Ajzen 1975; Ajzen and Fishbein 1980). If one includes beliefs, but replaces evaluations with importances, in the expectancy-value model, it is possible that empirical predictions of the model will be similar to the Σbe. But this has not been studied much (see Rosenberg 1956, who defined the evaluative component in the Σbe as the amount of satisfaction or dissatisfaction with an attribute of an object).

Bagozzi (1986) compared three versions of the Σbe, where evaluations were operationalized, respectively, with pleasant–unpleasant, good–bad, and subjective conditional approach–avoidance items. The latter measures asked respondents to indicate whether they would donate blood, given the occurrence of each of a number of specific consequences (for example fear of needles, worry about fainting, time constraints). Bagozzi argued that for certain attitudinal objects (in this case an action) where complex emotional and moral implications occur, neither affective (pleasant–unpleasant) nor moral (good–bad) evaluations should capture the motivational impetus of beliefs. Rather, the determinative evaluation was hypothesized to be the resultant of affective and moral evaluations, as captured by subjective conditional approach–avoidance responses. The findings showed that only subjective conditional approach–avoidance items combined multiplicatively with beliefs to influence global attitudes (see also Bagozzi 1989). Figure 2.2 summarizes the processes involved.

A related issue with respect to use of the standard good–bad measure of evaluations is the following. For some attitudinal objects, a person's moral and affective evaluations may be independent and even incongruent with

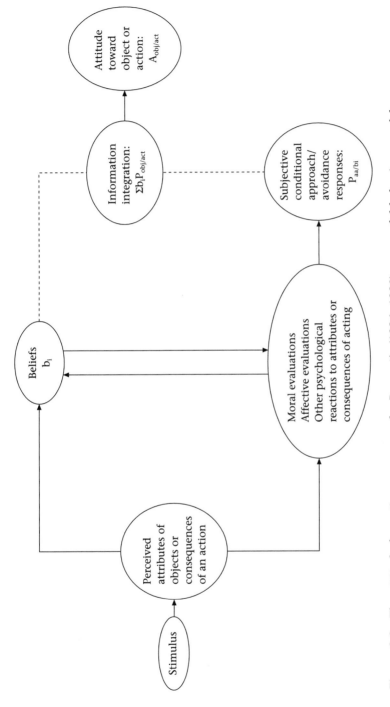

Figure 2.2 The attitude formation process under Bagozzi's (1986, 1989) purposeful behaviour model

Note: → equals causal relationship; ---- equals analytical relationship

each other and at the same time fail to correspond with the person's overall attitude. Some acts or consequences are emotionally repugnant, yet morally desirable (for example donating blood); others are affectively pleasing, yet ethically forbidden (for example extramarital sex); and still others coincide in both dimensions (for example attending church). To complicate matters, individuals may on occasion use a moral evaluation to downgrade or justify their own affective evaluation (or vice versa), depending on the context or their own dispositions. The good–bad measure captures moral connotations at best, yet can miss the mark for affective evaluations. Of course, things vary by circumstances, target object or act, and person. A good–bad reaction to a Burger King Whopper, for instance, could for one person reflect liking or disliking, for another a moral response (one may be a vegetarian or an animal rights activist), for still another a social reaction ('my group boycotts Burger King because it is a threat to my country, our cuisine, or family values concerning eating together at home') and for some people a utilitarian response ('eating beef increase my risk of heart disease'). We can see that the evaluative component of the expectancy-value model is a more complex issue than meets the eye. The approach suggested in Figure 2.2 is a fundamentally different perspective from the standard one and accommodates such complexities as mentioned above (Bagozzi 1986, 1989).

Functional form of the Σbe

Virtually all research conducted into expectancy-value models has focused on one form: the summation of the products of beliefs and evaluations. While this is an intuitive and parsimonious representation, other functional forms could be considered (Bagozzi 1985). In the interests of brevity, we shall limit comments here to the issue of additive versus averaging models, but it should be noted that many alternative functional forms could be investigated.

The Σbe is an additive model in the sense that it assumes that each belief is weighted or multiplied by a corresponding evaluation and the products are summed to yield an overall representation. The overall representation, depending on one's point of view, either represents a global attitude or is a distinct, unidimensional determinant of one's global attitude. One implication of the additive model is that the introduction of new information (for example a new product attribute) should either raise or lower one's attitude, depending on whether the information is positive or negative.

By contrast, the averaging model maintains that each belief and its corresponding evaluation is averaged to produce an overall representation. For example, one way to capture attitude through an averaging model is $A_{obj} = \Sigma b_i e_i^*$ where the constraint is imposed that $\Sigma e_i = 1$. The averaging model assumes that people form an attitude by integrating each belief more or less as a weighted average, where the weights are one's evaluations (Anderson 1981). The averaging model is also applied to the computation of one's global attitude at a point in time as a function of one's earlier, initial attitude, which is updated as new information becomes known. Notice that the averaging model does not necessarily imply that the introduction of a new piece of information will invariably increase an overall judgement if the information is positive or decrease it if it is negative, as required by the additive model described above. In fact, if a positive piece of information is added to another positive piece, and the former is of a lower magnitude than the latter, the averaging model would predict a decrease in the overall attitude. The opposite will happen for the parallel case where negative information is added to existing negative information: the overall attitude may increase, under the averaging model.

Which of the two approaches is more valid? Research showed early on that the averaging model performed better (for example Troutman and Shanteau 1976; Lynch 1979). However, Yamagishi and Hill (1981) demonstrated that the more favourable performance of the averaging model over the adding rests on the assumption of independence among the items of information (that is, independence among beliefs). Realistically, in most consumer decision contexts, beliefs will not be independent and in fact are typically moderately to highly correlated. Yamagishi and Hill (1981) found that an additive model performed best when the assumption of independence is relaxed.

The debate between additive and adding approaches has been in one sense wide of the mark. For one thing, many researchers in this debate have taken attitude (or more commonly, judgement has been studied) to be defined as the sum or average of weighted information. But attitude researchers more frequently consider attitude and the Σbe to be distinct, but interrelated, constructs. Under this point of view, it is possible to represent A_{obj} and the Σbe as separate latent variables and have multiple manifest measures of each as indicators. This specification uses what is known as structural equation models to represent the relationship. We will not consider the statistical model and issues here, and the reader is referred to the literature (for example Bagozzi 1980, 1994c). Under this representation, the latent expectancy-value construct can predict or be predicted by the latent global attitude construct. Each measure of the expectancy-value construct needs to be highly corre-lated with the other co-measures (this is implied by the requirement of unidimensionality; we will discuss later the case where beliefs are not all highly correlated, when multidimensional attitudes are treated). Each exist-ing measure (and each new measure added later, if any) for the expectancy-value construct is, in effect, part of the average of measures, if we were to focus on the factor mean of the latent variable for purposes of compar-isons across samples or groups of consumers, say. But each expectancy-value measure is related linearly to the single latent expectancy-value construct. In sum, the model of most relevance to attitude researchers hypothesizes that $A_{obj}^L = (\Sigma be)^L$, where the 'L' is included to stress that we have latent variables in mind. Another approach is to view A_{obj} as a linear function of $b_1 e_1, b_2 e_2, \ldots$, where each $b_i e_i$ is a separate independent variable. The above models and others are discussed in Bagozzi (1984, 1985; see also Bagozzi 1982).

Discussion of the functional form of the Σbe would not be complete without mention of the issue of what exactly does the construct depict. From our point of view, we might think of the Σbe as a representation of the information processing a consumer experiences when forming an attitude. That is, the Σbe represents the formation of beliefs and evaluations and integration of these into a summary form. Another meaning of the Σbe is as a representation of an attitude or the bases for an attitude which is stored in human memory and later retrieved or 'used' in decision making. Both of the above perspectives probably stretch things a bit, as it is unlikely that the Σbe captures what actually goes on in the minds of consumers. At best, the Σbe is an imperfect proxy or convenient tool for predicting global attitudes and other variables.

From another perspective, the Σbe might be construed as a summary of the processes that consumers go through to form an attitude. This, then, points to the need to give greater consideration to attitude formation and change processes. The elaboration likelihood model discussed in Chapter 5 is one such process model. Indeed, many of the processes discussed under the cognitive paradigm might be considered determinants of attitudes. We will present a sketch of still another basis for the Σbe later, when we discuss means-end chain theory. But first we have one more unresolved issue to discuss concerning expectancy-value models.

A scaling and statistical issue

The final unresolved issue we wish to consider with respect to the expectancy-value model pertains to the way the model is tested in statistical analyses. Naively, perhaps, the model is frequently applied as it appears: corresponding beliefs and evaluations, as measured, are multiplied times each other and the individual products or sums of products are treated as independent variables predicting A_{obj}. This practice, which is nearly universal, creates a serious problem in tests of hypotheses. Unless the measures of beliefs and evaluations are ratio-scaled, any tests of the effects of the products of beliefs and evaluations in the above sense will be arbitrary and uninterpretable (Cohen 1978; Bagozzi 1984; Evans 1991). Ratio scales are those such that ratios of scale values on measures correspond to ratios of values of the attributes. By design and in practice, measures of beliefs and evaluations are interval at best. As a consequence, it turns out that if one's measures are ordinal or interval, it is necessary to test the effects of product terms, while partialling out the main effects (that is, the separate effects of beliefs and evaluations). We agree with Eagly and Chaiken (1993: 235) that, when such tests are performed and the interaction is non-significant (that is, the products of beliefs and evaluations do not influence A_{obj}), it is not theoretically meaningful to interpret the main effects (because the psychological theory behind expectancy-value models does not support effects for beliefs on A_{obj} and for evaluations on A_{obj}). It would be an error, however, to suppose that a finding of a significant effect of, say, $b_i e_i$ on A_{obj} does not reflect a test of the theory proposed under expectancy-value theory, when main effects are partialled out. Indeed, this is the only valid test of the theory when measures are at best interval in nature. Tests of hypotheses between the sum of products of beliefs and evaluations and A_{obj}, when measures are at best interval, cannot be interpreted, if terms for beliefs and terms for evaluations are not included as additional independent variables. Unfortunately, the proper test has seldom been done, and the rationale behind it is frequently misconstrued (cf. Bagozzi 1984, 1986; Bagozzi and Warshaw 1990; Conner and McMillan 1999).

Problems with expectancy-value models and an appraisal-based alternative

In addition to scaling and statistical problems, expectancy-value models are limited in the sense that the summation of products of beliefs and evaluations obscures the differential influence, if any, of subsets of beliefs on attitudes. Instead, the expectancy-value model lumps all beliefs together in an undifferentiated whole. This practice not only clouds the explanatory power of the model (by failing to pinpoint the relative effects of beliefs), but also provides little practical guidance on what beliefs change agents should target.

Davis et al. (1989, 1992), in a study of the adoption of computer techno-logy, proposed and found that three fundamental beliefs or appraisals govern users' attitudes toward new programming technologies. Namely, adoption was found to be a function of perceived usefulness, ease of use, and fun in using the technologies. Rather than measuring beliefs and evaluations as specified under the expectancy-value model, Davis et al. suggested that con-sumers appraise the utilitarian, experiential, and enjoyment related conse-quences of adopting a product and these, in turn, govern one's overall attitude. This outlook is somewhat similar to research found in the literature on adoption of innovations where such factors as relative advantage and com-plexity of an innovation have been found to be particularly efficacious (for example Rogers 1995).

Gaither et al. (1997; see also Gaither et al. 1996) uncovered a broader set of appraisals governing attitudinal reactions in a study of physician use of drug information sources for therapeutic decision making. Specifically, it was found that physician attitudes toward one or more of seven sources of drug information depended on five appraisals: ease of use, usefulness, information quality on harmful effects, information quality on drug efficacy, and availabil-ity. Across the seven information sources (Physicians' Desk Reference, med-ical textbooks, medical journals/newsletters, pharmaceutical manufacturers' literature, pharmaceutical manufacturers' representatives, physician colleagues and pharmacists), the explained variance in attitudes ranged from 0.33 to 0.69, with usefulness the most important determinant and the other appraisals playing somewhat less, but generally important, roles, depending on the information source. For example, the most useful information source was pharmaceutical manufacturers' representatives, and the most important impact of information on harmful effects occurred for pharmacists as a source of information.

The main advantages of examining general appraisals, as opposed to expectancy-value determinants of attitudes, are parsimony, greater explanatory power and more informative policy recommendations. The approach provides fewer determinants and at the same time requires less time and effort to implement by use of questionnaires. One obtains a better sense of what exactly influences attitudes. And recommendations for changing attitudes are better grounded and more explicit. One thing that neither expectancy-value nor appraisal-based approaches do is to specify relationships among beliefs or among appraisals, if any, and their indirect and direct paths of influence on attitudes. We turn now to an approach that accomplishes what appraisal-based approaches accomplish but at the same time provides insights into the aetiology of reasons for developing a particular attitude and interrelationships among reasons.

Means-end chain theory

The expectancy-value model can be interpreted as an explanation for how attitudes develop. Namely, we develop our attitudes, in part, as a consequences of our beliefs and evaluations of beliefs concerning aspects of an attitudinal object or its implications for us. However, as detailed above, many unresolved issues can be identified with the expectancy-value model, so we might ask whether an alternative exists for discovering the determinants of attitudes (and such other abstract psychological representations as **desires, subjective norms, perceived behavioural control** and intentions). In addition to surmounting drawbacks with the expectancy-value model noted above, we would like to represent the determinants of attitudes and other abstract psychological constructs in a way capturing the underlying structure among beliefs and the causal, inferential, or functional relationships among beliefs, which the expectancy-value model does not do. Means-end chain theory is one approach that overcomes shortcomings of the expectancy-value model.

Means-end chain theory was originally developed for relating consumers' product knowledge to their self-knowledge (Gutman 1982; Olson and Reynolds 1983; Audenaert and Steenkamp 1997). Knowledge is presumed to be organized in a hierarchy with concrete thoughts linked to more abstract thoughts in a sequence progressing from *means* to *ends*. A threefold categorization of knowledge is presumed. Specifically, concrete knowledge about product attributes is connected to more abstract ideas about psychological and social consequences of the attributes, and the psychosocial consequences are, in turn, associated with even more abstract values (for example Reynolds and Gutman 1988). To take a specific example, one means-end chain for a sample of downhill skiers revealed the following sequence of inferences: ski packages → save money → ski more → fun and excitement → social atmosphere (Klenosky et al. 1993).

A number of procedures have been advocated for generating means-end chains. We adapted a procedure developed by Pieters et al. (1995) to derive a hierarchical structure of superordinate goals held by people desiring to lose or maintain their body weight. The hierarchical goal structure was generated by asking people to (1) provide reasons for their goal of losing/maintaining their body weight, (2) next supply justifications for each reason, and (3) give explanations for each justification (Bagozzi and Edwards 1998). Figure 2.3 presents the results for a sample of 197 men and women. We can think of this representation roughly as a cognitive schema; that is, it is a knowledge structure constituting the reasons for pursuing the goal of losing/maintaining body weight (Anderson 1980; Fiske and Taylor 1991). The basic units of this cognitive schema are superordinate goals to which the focal goal of losing/maintaining one's body weight is connected. By 'goal', we mean 'a mental image or other end point representation associated with affect toward which action may be directed' (Pervin 1989: 474). From one point of view,

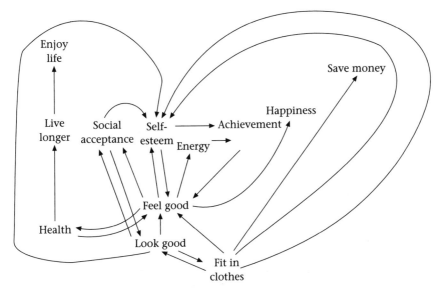

Figure 2.3   Hierarchical goal structure for reasons for losing or maintaining body weight

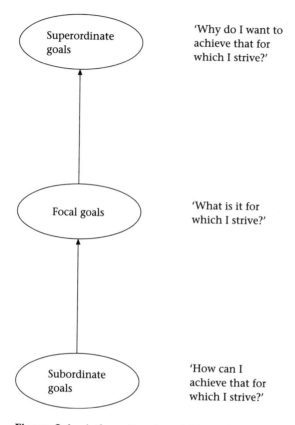

'Why do I want to achieve that for which I strive?'

'What is it for which I strive?'

'How can I achieve that for which I strive?'

Figure 2.4 A three-tiered goal hierarchy

the superordinate goals in Figure 2.3 are a type of 'declarative knowledge' in that they capture abstract, factual information (Anderson 1983). 'Happiness', 'self-esteem', 'feel good', etc. are abstract reasons for losing/maintaining weight. The linkages between superordinate goals are a type of 'procedural knowledge' in that they resemble if–then propositions (Anderson 1983): 'If I look good as a result of losing weight, I shall be accepted socially'. For an alternative interpretation of means-end theory, see Bagozzi and Dabholkar (2000) who view cognitive schemas as a 'grammar of discursive representations of oneself to oneself or to others' (Harré and Stearns 1995: 6).

To see how a cognitive schema of superordinate goals fits into a larger picture of decision making, see Figure 2.4, which can be considered an expanded goal hierarchy consisting of three fundamental tiers. A focal goal that one has (for example 'I want to lose three pounds over the next month') is located at the centre of the hierarchy and answers the question, 'What is it for which I strive?' Subordinate goals constitute the means of achieving the focal goal and answer the question, 'How can I achieve that for which I strive?' For the focal goal of losing three pounds, the subordinate goals might be various exercising and dieting routines. At the top of the hierarchy are superordinate goals, which answer the question, 'Why do I want to achieve that for which I strive?'. Figure 2.3 depicts a superordinate goal structure for losing/maintaining body weight. Researchers have proposed similar frameworks as shown in Figure 2.4 (for example Pieters 1993; Carver and Scheier 1998). Lawson (1997) showed how brand choice can be conceived as a function of a hierarchy of goals, beginning with abstract values that influence goals targeted toward product categories.

Hierarchical superordinate goal structures can be used to explain attitudes and such abstract psychological constructs as subjective norms. One way that this is done is to use multiple regression to show the dependence of attitudes on superordinate goals and the linkages between these goals. For example, Bagozzi and Edwards (1998) found that attitudes toward failing to lose/maintain body weight were a function of the superordinate goals, 'social acceptance' and 'self-esteem', as well as four linkages: 'health'→ 'live longer', 'health'→ 'achievement', 'health'→ 'energy' and 'fit in clothes'→ 'feel good'. Felt normative pressure to lose/maintain weight was found to be a function of one goal and eleven linkages.

We have shown that means-end chain theory can be applied to goals. It also has been applied to value structures concerning reactions to former US President Bill Clinton (Bagozzi and Dabholkar 2000) and motive structures related to joining or re-enlisting in the army (Bagozzi et al. 2001a).

Another way to look at how goals are represented in memory is by use of a category-based conceptualization. Barsalou (1991) argues that knowledge in the cognitive system is represented in categories, and there are two fundamental ways categories originate: through exemplar learning or conceptual combination. Exemplar learning is central to acquiring taxonomic knowledge about the world as it exists and is a relatively passive, bottom-up, and automatic process. Goal-derived categories, in contrast, are believed to arise through conceptual combination by manipulation of existing knowledge in memory. Barsalou (1991) summarizes aspects of categorization in this sense as follows:

Conceptual combination appears to be relatively active, top-down, and effortful. By deliberately manipulating knowledge through reasoning, people produce new categories that serve their goals . . . conceptual combination often produces idealized knowledge about how the world should be . . . rather than . . . about how it is.

(Barsalou 1991: 4)

Barsalou (1991: 27) further proposes that goals and their attributes are represented in *frames*, which he defines as 'flexible, loosely organized bodies of knowledge'. For example, the frame for a vacation goal might consist of the vacation category and its connections to five attributes: locations, temporal parameters, activities, objects and actors. Each attribute, in turn, might be connected to clusters of more specific attributes; for example, departure, duration, return and schedule are types of temporal parameters, and preparations, travel and entertainment are types of activities. The specific attributes further might be composed of subtypes; for example, major travel (flying transcontinentally), minor travel (taxi from airport to hotel) and arrangements at location (reserving a seat on a tour bus) are subtypes of travel. Barsalou (1991) shows how such frames are useful in planning goals and how other goals and constraints promote planning. For example, in planning a vacation, such background goals as 'maximize relaxation and educational value' guide the selection of exemplars for a frame instantiation. Within a particular frame, certain attributes also constrain the range of other attributes; for instance, a needed departure of July for a snow-skiing vacation requires a ski resort in the southern hemisphere. Much remains to be done in the study of the representation of consumer goals, but recent research and insights in memory for brands and attributes promises to deepen our understanding of goals (for example Bettman et al. 1998; Luce 1998).

Multidimensional models of attitude

Global attitudes and expectancy-value attitudes are perhaps most frequently thought to be unidimensional responses. But there are multidimensional models of global and expectancy-value attitudes as well. Before we consider these, it is helpful to discuss why multidimensional attitudes might exist. Some social psychologists have resisted the idea of multidimensionality, and indeed make sure in their research to construct unidimensional attitudes. They do this by applying specialized techniques in attitudinal scaling that guarantee unidimensionality. This of course precludes the chance in any study that the researcher will discover that respondents have multidimensional attitudes, if any. In other words, the practice of selecting items to measure a unidimensional attitude begs the question of whether attitudes can be multidimensional. If all we specify and measure are unidimensional attitudes, then multidimensionality is defined away.

But at least toward some objects and for some people, attitudes might be multidimensional. Multidimensionality can occur in at least two senses. An evaluative attitude toward an object might be formed and stored in memory as a set of distinct evaluations toward each of well-defined aspects of the object or its consequences for a person. The distinct evaluations could be unorganized or organized in a structure or network of interconnected subevaluations, either horizontally or perhaps hierarchically (see discussion below). Imagine, for example, that a new candidate for mayor announces their intentions to run for office. You do not know anything about the person or their qualifications, so you attend a public meeting where the candidates make known their positions and plans on issues and answer questions from perspective voters. By the end of the meeting, you may well form a number of evaluations toward various aspects of the candidate or issues on which the candidate stands but not necessarily have developed an overall evaluation one way or the other of the candidate. The multiple evaluations may be unrelated or may be loosely related without forming a singular attitude. In other instances, people may form multiple evaluations toward an object that remain distinct, have unique antecedents and produce unique consequences. This may be a result of the complexity of the object, the level of knowledge or expertise of the person, the cognitive style of the person, prior learning, and so on.

Another way that an attitude can be multidimensional is in terms of the nature and scope of its content. It is possible that attitudes are not limited to evaluative responses construed narrowly. Some researchers have maintained that attitudes have three components: cognitive (that is, beliefs or thoughts about an attitude object), affective (that is, emotions toward an object) and behavioural (that is, actions or behavioural responses) (for example Krech and Crutchfield 1948; Katz and Stotland 1959; Rosenberg and Hovland 1960). Tests of these components have confirmed this (for example Ostrom 1969; Kothandapani 1971; Bagozzi 1978), but as we develop later in the chapter, the tripartite model of attitude has little utility beyond historical or heuristic value, and more specific multidimensional conceptualizations are needed.

Multidimensional expectancy-value models

In a study of blood donors, Bagozzi (1981a, 1981b, 1982) found that beliefs (and by implication expectancy-value attitudes) about the negative consequences of giving blood formed three distinct components or dimensions: beliefs about immediate external pain (sore arm, hurts), immediate internal sickness (feel nauseated, lose consciousness) and delayed costs of a means-end variety (resistance lowered, lose time, curtail sports/exercise). Figure 2.5 shows the confirmatory factor analysis model used to represent the three distinct belief clusters about giving blood (Bagozzi 1994a: 340; see also Bagozzi 1981a, 1981b, 1982, where the structure is based on expectancy-value items and not merely beliefs).

Apparently, people conceive of giving blood as producing three well-defined, negative consequences (for a fourth cluster of beliefs concerning such positive consequences of giving blood as gaining a feeling of self-satisfaction, fulfilling a social obligation to help others, and ensuring an adequate blood supply for oneself and one's family and friends, see Bagozzi 1986: 100). Bagozzi (1981a) also found that the organization and structure of individual belief-evaluation products was the same as shown in Figure 2.5. In sum, rather than forming a singular expectancy-value reaction (that is, Σbe), people experience a multidimensional depiction of the consequences of giving blood in their minds. Multidimensional expectancy-value attitudes have also been

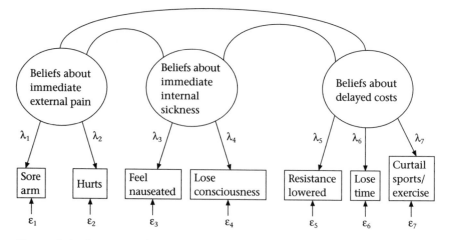

Figure 2.5 Structure of beliefs about the consequences of giving blood: confirmatory factor analysis representation (see Bagozzi 1994a: 340)

found by Oliver and Bearden (1985) in their study of the purchase of diet suppressants and by Shimp and Kavas (1984) in their study of coupon usage for products.

Given the possibility of multidimensional evaluations in the expectancy-value sense, it is interesting to ask what implications this has. Well, researchers are only now beginning to discover that the multiple dimensions can have distinct origins or causes, as well as distinct effects on other mental processes, decisions, or actions. We will have more to say on the causal role of attitudes in Chapter 4. For now, we wish only to suggest briefly the value of investigating multidimensional expectancy-value models. Figures 2.6 and 2.7 present two ways that overall attitude has been modelled as a function of multiple expectancy-value reactions. In Figure 2.6, A_{act} toward giving blood is shown to be a function of individual belief-evaluation products, organized according to the four dimensions alluded to above (see Bagozzi 1994a: 238). Here we have included additive terms for the separate evaluations and beliefs to control for the statistical indeterminacy in measurement for products of variables mentioned earlier (for example Bagozzi 1984). The main paths of interest in Figure 2.6 are marked as a, b, c and d, whereas the other paths impinging on A_{act} are solely for statistical control. This model was tested on data by means of partial least squares.

Figure 2.7 shows a similar model (with positive consequences omitted) for predicting overall attitude, where we have omitted error terms and factor loadings for simplicity (cf. Figure 2.5). This model hypothesizes that overall attitude occurs as a unidimensional dependent variable, and this, in turn, is influenced by a higher-order summary representation of expectancy-value attitudes. The summary expectancy-value attitude is portrayed with three

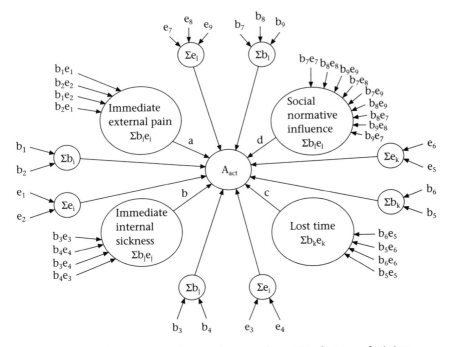

Figure 2.6 Multidimensional expectancy-value attitude toward giving blood with additive and multiplicative effects (see Bagozzi 1994a: 338)

dimensions. Because the left-off hand of Figure 2.7 is essentially the same as Figure 2.5, we have left off the verbal labels for measures of each dimension of the expectancy-value attitude for simplicity. Semantic differential labels for measures of A_{act} are provided (that is, 'good–bad' and so on). The difference between Figures 2.6 and 2.7 lies primarily in whether one construes expectancy-value attitudes as defined by belief-evaluation products or whether belief-evaluation products indicate or reflect expectancy-value attitudes. This issue concerns complex conceptual and operational issues that we will not address herein.

The final implication we wish to consider with regard to multidimensional expectancy-value models can best be conveyed through an example. Although advertising is often an effective way to change beliefs (or evaluations), some beliefs are difficult to change or are too sensitive to target for change. Sometimes it is necessary to single-out a particular belief (evaluation) by attacking another belief (evaluation) more vulnerable or acceptable to change efforts. Persuasive communication can be fine-tuned to influence a specific belief (evaluation) and then indirectly, through another belief (evaluation), affect attitude. The unidimensional expectancy-value model, being a singular agglomeration of beliefs and evaluations, provides little guidance on which

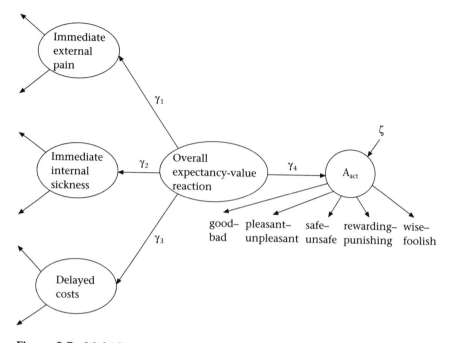

Figure 2.7 Multidimensional expectancy-value attitude toward giving blood – latent variable approach (see Bagozzi 1982)

beliefs or evaluations to target because it has nothing to say about interrelations or sequences among beliefs (Bagozzi 1981a).

Yi (1989) investigated the indirect effects of advertising on the network of beliefs and evaluations comprising a multidimensional expectancy-value attitude. Figure 2.8 summarizes the structure he examined in the context of an experimental study of consumer attitudes toward Hyundai automobiles. It was believed, and pre-tests showed, that favourable expectancy-value attitudes toward maintenance costs would be difficult to create, in part because the automobile was new and unknown and people at the time had sceptical attitudes toward Korean cars. But it was possible to create advertisements wherein favourable beliefs and evaluations concerning dependability or reliability were created in the minds of consumers. This was done through verbal arguments in one case and through the portrayal of role playing and vicarious learning in another. The findings showed that consumers inferred favourable levels of anticipated maintenance costs on the basis of information provided in the ads on dependability. Figure 2.8 shows how this happened (see path c). Multidimensional expectancy-value attitude models thus provide a better way to examine complex effects of advertising on consumer reactions than does the traditional Σbe approach.

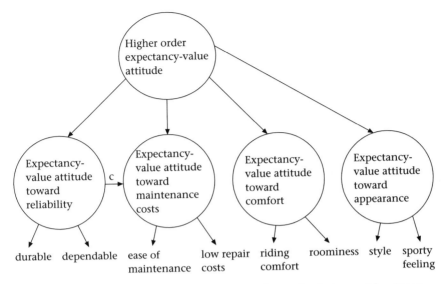

Figure 2.8 Multidimensional expectancy-value attitude toward buying a Hyundai automobile (based on Yi 1989)

Multidimensional representations of global attitudes

The affective-cognitive-behavioural model of attitude has received little currency in recent years. For one thing, researchers have shifted focus to the explanation of action and therefore have in a sense removed behaviour, per se, as a component of attitude, and come to see the remainder of whatever attitude represents as a determinant of behaviour. We shall return to this perspective in Chapter 4. This leaves the affective and cognitive components as candidates for a multidimensional conceptualization of attitude. Early work showed that affect and cognition can be separate dimensions and function differentially in the prediction of behaviour (for example Bagozzi and Burnkrant 1979; for a debate, see Bagozzi and Burnkrant 1985; Dillon and Kumar 1985). But little new has been done of late. One problem seems to be with the nature of the cognitive component. It is unclear whether cognitions, per se, can have emotive power or motivational content in the same way that affective variables do and in the sense we take the everyday meaning of attitude to imply. On the other hand, if we take the cognitive content of attitude to be a species of evaluation, it is unclear whether we gain anything by calling it cognitive.

Recently, researchers have shifted focus to a bicomponent perspective where affect and evaluations constitute two distinct, yet empirically associated, aspects of attitude. Note, however, that researchers have not been consistent in their use of terminology for the non-affective dimension. Sometimes they have used the word beliefs but employed evaluative items to measure it; at other times, the word cognitions is used but evaluations measured; and at still other times the word beliefs has been used to refer to the strength of connection between a target object and its affective characteristics.

Breckler and Wiggins (1989) studied various attitudinal targets. For example, they asked people in their Study 1 to 'indicate your beliefs' by rating 'blood donation' on five 7-point semantic differential scales (good–bad, wise–foolish, important–unimportant, unselfish–selfish, safe–unsafe) and to express how 'blood donation' 'makes you feel' on the same scales. The results showed that affect and evaluation correlated $r = 0.77$. In Study 2, Breckler and Wiggins (1989) found that the same affective and evaluative components correlated $r = 0.83$. In addition, separate measures by use of equal appearing interval scales revealed that affect and evaluations correlated only $r = 0.24$. In both studies, 'global attitude' was measured with a single 7-point, like–dislike item. This item correlated $r = 0.64$ and $r = 0.63$ with affect and evaluations, respectively, in Study 1; $r = 0.57$ and $r = 0.36$ with affect and evaluation measures, respectively, and $r = 0.57$ and $r = 0.29$ with the equal appearing interval affect and evaluation measures, respectively, in Study 2. A limitation of their study is that the measure of global attitude is an affective measure, not an evaluative one, and at the same time taps only one sense of affect (that is, love–hate) while neglecting others (for example happy–sad, fearful–calm, aroused–unaroused).

Eagly et al. (1994) investigated attitudes toward social groups and policies. In Study 1, reactions toward women, men, Democrats and Republicans were measured. Overall attitude was indicated by responses to five 7-point semantic differential items (good–bad, positive–negative, valuable–useless, pleasant–unpleasant and nice–awful), beliefs were measured by estimates of the strength of association between each target group and up to ten self-generated characteristics (for example 'friendly') and affect was recorded by asking subjects to generate up to ten emotions they typically felt toward the members of the respective groups. The findings showed that beliefs and affect correlated $r = 0.22 - 0.62$ across the four target groups. In addition, regression of overall attitude on both beliefs and affect demonstrated that beliefs were significant predictors across all four target groups, but affect was significant only for Republicans. In Study 2, similar procedures were used to measure reactions toward abortion on demand, affirmative action in employment, and welfare. The results revealed that beliefs and affect correlated $r = 0.50 - 0.60$ across issues; beliefs significantly predicted each issue in regression analyses, but affect only predicted abortion.

Crites et al. (1994) investigated reactions toward literature, maths, capital punishment, birth control, church and snakes by use of a variety of scaling techniques (semantic differential, multi-response checklist, dichotomous checklist, word variation). The findings supported distinct affective and cognitive (that is, evaluative) factors. Across the six issues, affect and evaluation correlated $r = 0.27 - 0.86$ and predicted overall attitude in most cases. In a somewhat similar study, Trafimow and Sheeran (1998) found that cognitive and affective beliefs achieved convergent and discriminant validity (the factors correlated $r = 0.48$ and $r = 0.16$ in their experiments 1 and 2, respectively).

One limitation of the aforementioned studies is that they scrutinized affective and evaluative *bases* (that is, antecedents) of unidimensional global attitudes and did not measure overall attitude in separate affective and evaluative senses. In contrast, Ajzen and Driver (1991) report evidence for separate affective and evaluative components of A_{act} in their study of leisure activities. Bagozzi et al. (2001b) found separate affective and evaluative attitudes toward the act of donating bone marrow, and this occurred in four samples: Chinese in Hong Kong, Chinese Americans in San Francisco, and African American and white Americans in Ann Arbor, Michigan. Affective A_{act} was measured with enjoyable–unenjoyable, pleasant–unpleasant, comfortable–uncomfortable, attractive–unattractive and appealing–unappealing items; evaluative A_{act} was measured with rewarding–punishing, wise–foolish, beneficial–harmful, useful–useless and good–bad items. Bagozzi et al. (2001b) found that affective and evaluative attitudes predicted decision making to different degrees, once multi-collinearity was taken into account.

It might be concluded, based on the emerging research reviewed above, that global attitudes show two components – affective and evaluative – and the components can be dependent on different antecedents and predict consequences differentially. Fishbein (1993: xxiii) offers a caution, however: 'one should ask whether one wants multiple attitude measures or if these different measures are best viewed as indicants of a single attitudinal construct that captures all possible meanings of "good/bad" [that is, evaluation] and/or "like/dislike" [that is, affect]'. Indeed, Bagozzi et al. (2001b) showed that the separate evaluative and affective responses for A_{act} could be organized as two first-order factors and comprised two dimensions of a single higher-order factor in a confirmatory factor analysis model. In other words, there are distinct affective and evaluative attitudinal responses at one level of abstraction, but these are accounted for by an overall attitude at a still higher level of abstraction. We see, then, that attitude is both multidimensional and unidimensional, depending on what level of analysis we study it.

Multidimensionality and goal-directed attitudes

This brings us to our final issue concerning multidimensionality. Eagly and Chaiken (1993: 13) suggest that the empirical separability of components of attitude is interesting as far as it goes, but we should perhaps be more concerned about identifying the circumstances under which multidimensionality occurs (see also Breckler 1984). One of the few areas to date that this point of view has been taken is in research on goal-directed attitudes.

Up to this point, we have taken the classic interpretation of attitude which sees it as 'a psychological tendency that is expressed by evaluating a particular entity with some degree of favor or disfavor' (Eagly and Chaiken 1993: 1). The psychological tendency embodied by an attitude is sometimes termed an acquired behavioural disposition (Campbell 1963). As such, attitudes are automatic evaluative responses to an object. Moreover, the acquisition of an attitude is thought to be primarily through learning or conditioning.

But attitudes toward acts that are perceived to be problematic in the eyes of a decision maker (because, for example, one lacks needed resources or the situation contains impediments to successful implementation of goal-directed behaviours) are formed in fundamentally different ways than dispositional attitudes. Bagozzi and Warshaw (1990) proposed that decision makers come to see such acts from the point of view of **trying** to act. For example, to lower one's blood pressure, patients may see their task as trying to do the things needed to accomplish this goal: taking medication regularly, reducing salt intake, eating healthily, exercising, refraining from smoking or drinking alcoholic beverages, and coping with stress. Motivation and commitment

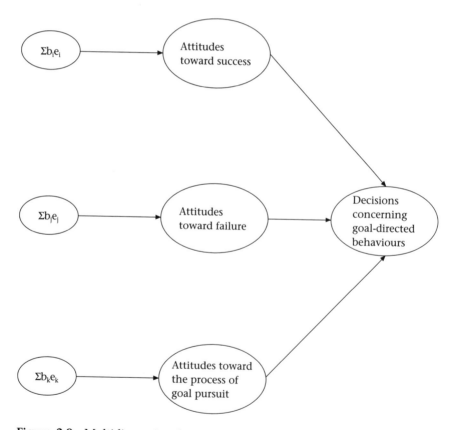

Figure 2.9 Multidimensional attitudes and their role in decision making concerning goal-directed behaviours

must be marshalled, temptations resisted, and impediments overcome to implement these instrumental acts.

In such situations, Bagozzi and Warshaw (1990) suggested that attitudes form in three distinct dimensions. Two of these dimensions refer specifically to the *outcomes* of goal attainment: namely, trying to reach a goal and *succeeding* (attitudes toward success) and trying to reach a goal and *failing* (attitudes toward failure). Similarly, separate from outcomes of success and failure, decision makers appraise the means or *processes* leading up to goal attainment or not (attitudes toward the process). Figure 2.9 shows the three attitudinal components, where each is modelled as a function of its own unique expectancy-value reactions and each influences decisions concerning goal-directed behaviours. Bagozzi and Warshaw's (1990) original **theory of trying** also included expectations of success and expectations of failure, which interacted with attitudes toward success and failure, respectively, to influence decision, but these are omitted here for simplicity (see discussion of theory of trying Chapter 4).

A growing body of research supports the model shown in Figure 2.9. This research covers such topics as regulating hypertension (Taylor et al. 2001), studying for exams (Leone and Perugini 2000), adopting new computer technologies (Bagozzi et al. 1992c), low-risk single-occasion drinking (Murgraff et al. 2000), exercising and dieting (Bagozzi and Kimmel 1995), losing weight (Bagozzi and Warshaw 1990; Bagozzi and Edwards 1998), achieving goals in experimental tasks (Hinsz and Ployhart 1998) and diet or dieting decisions (Bagozzi et al. 2001c; Capozza and Bagozzi 2001).

Conclusion

We have seen that attitudes are evaluative and/or affective responses to objects. The expectancy-value model is a leading unidimensional perspective on attitudes and maintains that attitudes are based on, or determined by, the product of beliefs and evaluations of attributes of objects. This model has been applied frequently in consumer research because of its policy implications for attitude change. A number of unresolved issues with the expectancy-value model were discussed. The chapter also investigated multidimensional attitudes, which were shown to exist in expectancy-value and affective-evaluative structures. In the next chapter, we introduce emotions and their role in consumer behaviour. This is followed by a chapter which integrates attitudes and emotions, with other variables, to explain consumer action.

Suggested readings

Bagozzi, R.P. and Edwards, E.A. (1998) Goal setting and goal pursuit in the regulation of body weight, *Psychology and Health*, 13: 593–621. Part 2 of this article develops a more general laddering procedure that applies to abstract outcomes and goals, as well as products and services, and uses it to illustrate the case of body weight management.

Bagozzi, R.P. and Warshaw, P.R. (1990) Trying to consume, *Journal of Consumer Research*, 17: 127–40. Derives a three-dimensional model of attitudes toward goals (attitudes toward success, failure, and process), introduces the concept trying, and specifies two aspects of past behaviour effects (frequency and recency).

Barsalou, L.W. (1991) Deriving categories to achieve goals, in G.H. Bower (ed.) *The Psychology of Learning and Motivation*, vol. 27. New York: Academic Press. Shows how goal-derived categories arise through conceptual combination by manipulation of existing knowledge.

Eagly, A.H. and Chaiken, S. (1993) *The Psychology of Attitudes*. Fort Worth, TX: Harcourt Brace Jovanovich. The most comprehensive treatment of attitude theory and related areas from social psychology. A classic.

Fishbein, M. and Ajzen, I. (1975) *Belief, Attitude, Intention, and Behavior: An Introduction to Theory and Research*. Reading, MA: Addison-Wesley. Presents the early history of attitudes in social psychology and is especially useful for describing expectancy-value models.

Reynolds, T.J. and Gutman, J. (1988) Laddering theory, method, analysis and interpretation, *Journal of Advertising Research*, 28: 11–31. Develops the procedure for applying the laddering technique wherein attributes→psychosocial consequences→values. Particularly applicable to physical products but can be adapted to services.

3

Consumers are emotional, too

The social psychology of consumer behaviour, like its parent discipline, social psychology, has been rooted in cognition, which philosophers define as 'the domain of representational states and processes . . . involved in thinking . . . using a language, guiding and controlling behaviour' (Honderich 1995: 138). Philosophers distinguish between cognition, on the one hand, and sensations (for example pain), perceptions, and feelings or emotions, on the other hand. Until relatively recently, researchers have neglected emotional aspects of consumer behaviour. In this chapter, we explore the role of emotions in consumer behaviour and review extant research (see also Bagozzi et al. 1999a).

Theory and function of emotions

Little consistency can be found in the use of terminology related to emotions. For purposes of organization and discussion, we begin with a definition of emotions and then turn to a framework for interpreting emotional behaviour.

Definitions

The term *affect* can be conceived as an umbrella for a set of more specific mental processes including emotions, **moods** and (possibly) attitudes. Thus, affect might be considered a general category for mental feeling processes, rather than a particular psychological process, per se.

By emotion, we mean a mental state of readiness that arises from cognitive appraisals of events or thoughts, has a phenomenological tone, is accompanied by physiological processes, is often expressed physically (for example in gestures, posture, facial features) and may result in specific actions to affirm or cope with the emotion, depending on its nature and meaning for the person having it (see also Lazarus 1991; Oatley 1992).

The line between an emotion and mood is frequently difficult to draw, but often by convention involves conceiving of a mood as being longer lasting (from a few hours up to days) and lower in intensity than an emotion. Yet, exceptions can be found. Still another distinction between emotions and moods is that the former typically is intentional (that is, it has an object or referent), whereas moods are generally nonintentional and global or diffused (Frijda 1993). Also, moods are not as directly coupled with **action tendencies** and explicit actions as are many emotions.

Finally, attitudes, too, are often considered instances of affect, with the same measures used on occasion to indicate emotions and attitudes (for example pleasant–unpleasant, happy–sad or interested–bored semantic differential items). However, some authors take a narrower view of attitudes and define them as evaluative judgements (measured, for example, by good–bad reactions) rather than emotional states. Cohen and Areni (1991), for instance, reserve the term affect for 'valenced feeling states', with emotions and moods as specific examples. Attitudes are evaluative judgements in their view. Nevertheless, other researchers do not make a distinction between affect and evaluative judgements. See our discussions in Chapter 2 where it was noted that many psychologists have equated affect with evaluation, yet in recent years, other researchers have shown that affective and evaluative attitudes are distinct.

It should be recognized that the terms *affect, emotions, moods* and *attitudes* have frequently been used inconsistently in the literature. When reading the literature, it is important to pay attention to both how authors define affective (and related) terminologies and how they measure the variables to which the terminologies refer. One's definition of terms permits an interpretation of their meaning but equally important is how the variables to which the terms refer are operationalized. Some authors have defined key variables as emotions, moods or attitudes but have used operationalizations corresponding to different concepts. Other authors have used operationalizations for a single variable that cut across two or more instances of affect. To make clear our definition of emotions and how it differs from definitions of mood and attitudes, we present the following point of view.

Organizing framework

Above we noted that emotions are mental states of readiness. But so, too, are moods and attitudes. How then might we distinguish among these affective states? For one thing, the state of readiness characterized by an emotion tends to be more intense than that characterized by moods or attitudes. It is more intense in the sense of strength of felt subjective experience, plus magnitude of physiological response (for example autonomic nervous system activity) and extent of bodily expression (for example facial displays), when these latter reactions accompany an emotion.

Probably the most important factor differentiating emotions from moods and attitudes is the way emotions arise. Emotions are said to have a specific referent (for example a consumer becomes pleased when a new detergent removes grass stains from clothing; someone is angered by poor service in a restaurant). More specifically, emotions arise in response to appraisals one makes for something of relevance to one's well-being. By appraisal, we mean an assessment and interpretation thereof. By something of relevance, we mean an incident or episode that happens to oneself (for example an unplanned event), a behaviour one performs or a result one produces (for example engaging in an activity or receiving or failing to receive a planned outcome) or a change in an object, person or thought that has personal meaning for the self.

It is important to stress that, although categories of events or physical circumstances are frequently associated with particular emotional responses, it is not the specific events or physical circumstances that produce the emotions but rather the unique psychological appraisal made by the person assessing and interpreting the events and circumstances. Different people can have different emotional reactions (or no emotional reactions at all) to the same event or happening. Note, too, that appraisals can be deliberative, purposive and conscious, but also unreflective, automatic, and unconscious, depending on the person and eliciting conditions for emotional arousal. The central role of appraisals in the formation of emotions has come to define what are aptly called appraisal theories in psychology (for example Smith and Ellsworth 1985; Frijda 1986; Ortony et al. 1988; Lazarus 1991; Roseman 1991).

Appraisal theorists maintain that the critical determinant of any emotion is the resultant judgement and interpretation that arises after comparing an actual state to a desired state. Two appraisals are particularly crucial at this stage of emotion formation: goal relevance and goal congruence (Lazarus 1991). That is, a necessary condition for an emotional response to an event or happening is that a person has a personal stake in it and at the same time judges the event or happening to facilitate or thwart this stake.

A distinctive feature of appraisal theories is their specification of the conditions leading to discrete emotional responses. We focus on Roseman's (1991) version of appraisal theories, which differs in relatively minor ways from other leading theories. Roseman (1991) hypothesized that particular combinations of 5 appraisals determine which of 16 unique emotions will be experienced in any given situation. Figure 3.1 summarizes his theory, where the 5 appraisals are labelled motive-consistent/motive-inconsistent (that is, positive emotions versus negative emotions), appetitive/aversive (that is, presence of a reward versus absence of a punishment), agency (that is, outcome is perceived caused by impersonal circumstances, some other person, or the self), probability (that is, an outcome is certain or uncertain) and power (that is, strong versus weak coping potential).

For example, pride occurs when one evaluates one's own performance of an action or achievement of an outcome in a positive light (for example a

Circumstance caused	Positive emotions motive-consistent		Negative emotions motive-inconsistent		
	Appetitive	Aversive	Appetitive	Aversive	
unexpected	Surprise				
uncertain	Hope		Fear		Weak
certain	Joy	Relief	Sadness	Distress, disgust	Weak
uncertain	Hope		Frustration		Strong
certain	Joy	Relief	Frustration		Strong
other-caused uncertain	Liking		Dislike		Weak
certain	Liking		Dislike		Weak
uncertain	Liking		Anger		Strong
certain	Liking		Anger		Strong
self-caused uncertain	Pride		Shame, guilt		Weak
certain	Pride		Shame, guilt		Weak
uncertain	Pride		Regret		Strong
certain	Pride		Regret		Strong

(Left vertical label: Agency; right vertical label: Power)

Figure 3.1   Roseman's (1991) appraisal theory of emotions

Source: Roseman (1991: 193), reprinted with permission

feeling of having done well). Here the positive emotion is motive-consistent, either appetitive (for example having attained a positive goal) or aversive (for example having avoided a punishment), self-produced under weak or low coping potential, and either certain or uncertain, depending upon the circumstances. Sadness happens when one experiences a loss for which one recognizes that nothing can be done to restore it. The loss, which is of something or someone valued, is experienced negatively and with high certainty under conditions of low coping power. It is perceived to be caused by impersonal circumstances.

One value of appraisal theories is that it is possible to account for most emotions. Indeed, subtle combinations of appraisals yield discrete emotional responses. Anger and regret, for example, differ primarily in only one type of appraisal and share in the other four: namely, anger occurs when a person sees another person as the source of injury to oneself or to another person viewed as a victim of injustice, whereas regret results when one's negative outcome is attributed to actions or inactions of the self.

Not every emotion is accounted for by Roseman's framework (or by any other framework for that matter). For instance, pride is regarded as a positive emotion in Roseman's framework, yet excessive or exaggerated pride (sometimes termed *hubris*) can invite retribution. Likewise, shame and guilt are thought by Roseman to be produced by similar appraisals, but other researchers have found important distinctions among shame, guilt and embarrassment (for example Lewis 1993). Likewise, disgust has been studied extensively and found to differ from distress (for example Rozin et al. 1993). Nevertheless, in contrast to other theories of emotion which conceive of it in bipolar terms (for example pleasure–displeasure and high arousal–low arousal (Russell 1980) or high negative affect–low negative affect and high positive affect–low positive affect: Watson and Tellegen 1985), Roseman's framework and other appraisal theories not only allow for many discrete emotions but also specify conditions for their occurrence.

An elaboration of appraisal theories that is especially relevant for consumer behaviour is the treatment of *goals*, which may be defined as 'internal representations of desired states, where states are broadly defined as outcomes, events, or processes' (Austin and Vancouver 1996: 338). Oatley and Johnson-Laird (1987) proposed what they termed a *communicative theory of emotions* wherein events are evaluated in relation to a person's goals. Emotions are thought to function to coordinate parts of one's cognitive system so as to manage responses to events and in so doing change from ongoing to new activities or to maintain desired states or activities. The self-regulation of goals is believed to be the main function of emotions:

> Each goal and plan has a monitoring mechanism that evaluates events relevant to it. When a substantial change in probability occurs of achieving an important goal or subgoal, the monitoring mechanism broadcasts to the whole cognitive system a signal that can set it into readiness to respond to this change. Humans experience these signals and the states of readiness they induce as emotions.
>
> (Oatley 1992: 50)

According to Oatley and Johnson-Laird (1987: 35), emotions are evoked 'at a significant juncture of a plan . . . typically . . . when the evaluation (conscious or unconscious) of the likely success of a plan changes'. Positive emotions (for example happiness, elation, joy) are associated with the attainment of a (sub)goal, which usually leads to a decision to continue with the plan, whereas negative emotions (for example frustration, disappointment, anxiety) result from problems with ongoing plans and failures to achieve desired goals (see also Stein et al. 1996; Bagozzi et al. 1998).

Emotions have implications for action and goal attainment. Lazarus (1991) identifies **coping responses** as important mechanisms in this regard. When we experience a negative emotion (for example anger, sadness, fear), we are in disequilibrium and wish to return to our normal state. Either one or both of two coping processes are typically used: problem-focused coping, where we attempt to alleviate the sources of distress, or emotion-focused coping, where we either change the meaning of the source of distress (for example deny that a threat exists; distance oneself from the source of distress) or avoid thinking about a problem.

By contrast, coping with positive emotions often involves sharing one's good fortune, savoring the experience, working to continue or increase the rewards, and increasing physical activity. Positive emotions are sometimes accompanied as well by higher levels of physiological arousal, expanded **attention**, increased optimism, enhanced recall, and a shift from self- to other-centred orientations (for example becoming friendlier, caring about others), when compared, say, to sadness. Indeed, positive emotions, particularly happiness, frequently stimulate helping or altruistic actions. Why? Schaller and Cialdini (1990: 284–5) offer two explanations: 'First, we may propose that positive mood leads to enhanced helping via the more positive outlook and enhanced activity that appear to spring automatically from the experience of happiness', and second, 'we argue that happiness is associated with a motivation toward disequilibrium – toward the possible attainment of additional personal rewards that transcend the basic concern over one's mood'. The personal rewards referred to here concern such self-enrichment motives as affiliation, achievement, competence, and esteem.

Closely related to coping responses are action tendencies. An action tendency is 'a readiness to engage in or disengage from interaction with some goal object' and includes '[i]mpulses of "moving towards", "moving away", and "moving against"' (Frijda et al. 1989: 213). Some theorists maintain that emotions not merely are reactions to appraisals of events but also include action tendencies as part of their meaning (Frijda 1986). Others go further and maintain that action tendencies are automatic, 'pre-wired' responses connected to emotions (LeDoux 1996). In Frijda's (1986) treatment, emotions are conceived as the entire process from stimulus event to action and arousal:

Stimulus event→event coding→appraisal (evaluation of relevance, context

and urgency/difficulty/seriousness of event) →action readiness$\big\langle\begin{smallmatrix}\text{action}\\\text{arousal}\end{smallmatrix}$

Much as emotions arise in response to patterns of appraisals, Frijda (1986; Frijda et al. 1989) has shown that patterns of action readiness correspond to distinct emotion categories (for example avoidance with fear, helping with caring, helplessness with sadness, assault with anger, withdrawal with shame).

Finally, it has been argued that many coping responses to emotions are volitional (Bagozzi 1992: 186–9; Mick and Fournier 1998). The process begins with outcome–desire units and appraisals of changes or anticipated changes in goal attainment or goal progress. Four appraisal classes can be identified. *Outcome–desire conflicts* happen when one fails to achieve a goal or when one experiences an unpleasant event. One or more emotional reactions occur to outcome–desire conflicts (for example dissatisfaction, anger, shame, guilt, sadness, disappointment, disgust, regret), depending on attributions of the source of goal failure or the unpleasant event (that is, self, other person or external cause). The coping response(s) to these emotions, in turn, is selected from the following: intent to remove or undo harm, obtain help or support, decrease outcome, re-evaluate goal, or redouble effort, if appropriate, depending on the specific emotion involved.

Outcome–desire fulfilments take place when one achieves a goal, experiences a pleasant event or avoids an unpleasant event. One or more emotional reactions come about when outcome–desire fulfilments happen (for example satisfaction, joy, elation, pleasure, pride, relief, caring, love), again depending on attributions of the source of good fortune. The coping response(s) to these emotions include an intention to maintain, increase, share or enjoy the outcome.

Outcome–desire conflicts and fulfilments refer to outcomes in the past or present. The following two appraisal classes go on with regard to planned outcomes. *Outcome–desire avoidances* transpire in anticipation of unpleasant outcomes or goals. Fear or its variants (for example worry, anxiety, distress) are the emotional reactions to this appraisal. The coping response(s) to these emotions entail either an intention to avoid undesirable outcomes or to reinterpret the threat.

The final class of appraisals, *outcome–desire pursuits*, happen in anticipation of pleasant goals or outcomes. Hope is the emotional reaction to such appraisals. The coping response(s) to hope includes intentions to realize or facilitate outcome attainment and to sustain one's commitment and vigilance.

The **theory of self-regulation** suggests that unique volitional responses underlie coping for each particular emotion or class of emotions (Bagozzi 1992). In addition, the specific intention enacted depends on one's degree of **self-efficacy** in executing the coping responses. Somewhat analogous (appraisal → emotional reactions → coping) responses occur for outcome–identity conflicts, fulfilments, avoidances and pursuits in social situations related to normative expectations (Bagozzi 1992: 191–4).

Returning to the distinction between emotions and moods and attitudes, we might say that, in addition to the things mentioned earlier, emotions differ from moods and attitudes in the manner in which they arise and in their representation in memory. Emotions occur in response to changes in specific plans or goal-relevant events. As Oatley (1992: 64, 91–2) points out, emotions are manifest as 'transitions from one sequence of action and another', but moods occur 'when the cognitive system is maintained in an emotion mode for a period'. Indeed, moods are often resistant to changes in events surrounding them. One reason for this is that moods 'depend on the dissociability of control emotion signals from semantic information about causation' (Oatley 1992: 64). In general, moods are elicited by

(a) after effects of emotions; (b) organismic conditions such as illness, fatigue, previous exercise, and good health, or pharmacological agents; (c) general environmental conditions and side effects of activities: heat, noise, environmental variety, stressful conditions.

(Frijda 1986: 289)

Like emotions, attitudes can arise from changes in events, but attitudes also occur in response to mundane objects. In addition, arousal is a necessary part of emotions but not necessarily attitudes. Moreover, attitudes seem to have the capacity to be stored over long periods of time and retrieved, whereas emotions are not experienced in this way (that is, emotions are ongoing states of readiness; they are not stored and retrieved, per se, although it is possible to recreate the conditions originally producing them in our memory and react emotionally to the thoughts so generated, at least up to a point; emotions can, however, be classically conditioned, but it is unclear whether attitudes can). Finally, the connection of emotions to **volition** and action is stronger and more direct than it is for attitudes. Emotions directly stimulate volitions and initiate action, but attitudes may require an additional motivation impetus, such as desire (Bagozzi 1992; see also Chapter 4 in this book).

Measurement of emotions

The measurement of emotions could focus on a full set of signs or evidence, including evaluative appraisals, subjective feelings, body posture and gestures, facial expressions, physiological responses, action tendencies and overt actions. Whatever measurements one uses should, of course, be tied to an underlying theory of emotions.

Some authors (for example most appraisal theorists) construe emotions as mental states or processes, and thus it would be prudent to directly measure the cognitive activities comprising the emotional content of these states or processes, from this perspective. Self-reports of one's subjective experiences constitute the most frequently used procedures in this regard, although other methods for indicating emotional memory processes might be used as well (for example response time, subliminal **priming**). From the point of view of mental conceptualizations of emotions, physiological, motor or biological indicators would be at best considered correlates or indirect measures of emotions.

Other researchers who interpret emotions in broader terms, as either the whole process from the coding of events to action responses (for example Frijda 1986) or as complex patterns of physiological responses (for example Cacioppo et al. (1992a), maintain that emotional experience is a function of somatovisceral activation, afferentiation and cognitive operations; LeDoux (1996) emphasizes brain processes, especially the role of the **amygdala**) stress the need for measurement processes going beyond self-reports. Depending on the theorist, overt behaviours or physiological reactions may be considered either a part of what it means to have an emotion or antecedents, concomitants or possibly even effects of an emotion. More behaviourally or physiologically oriented researchers obviously employ measures of emotions consistent with these interpretations.

Consumer researchers have tended to take an empirical approach to the measurement of emotions and to rely on self-reports (that is, either unipolar or bipolar items on questionnaires). In the typical application, many items cutting across numerous positive and negative emotions are administered to measure reactions to a stimulus, and such methods as factor analysis, multidimensional scaling or cluster analysis are used to identify the underlying emotional dimensions for the sample at hand. The number of items investigated in this regard has been as large as 180 (Aaker et al. 1988), while a paper and pencil technique (basically a single item measured continuously while viewing an ad) has even been suggested to register 'warmth' toward a stimulus ad (Aaker et al. 1986; see also Russell et al. 1989).

Two influential studies in the measurement of emotional responses toward advertisements are those by Edell and Burke (1987) and Holbrook and Batra (1987). Edell and Burke (1987; see also Burke and Edell 1989) developed a 52-item scale for measuring emotions towards ads, while Holbrook and Batra (1987) worked with a 94-item scale, which was later reduced to 34 items (Batra and Holbrook 1990).

With so many items measuring emotions, a question arises whether a small number of basic dimensions underlie people's responses. Edell and Burke (1987) analysed the items in their scale and found three factors: upbeat feelings, negative feelings and warm feelings. Likewise, Holbrook and Batra (1987) used factor analysis, but in a slightly different way. Their 94 items were first generated a priori to measure 29 emotional indices. For example, joyful, happy, delighted and pleased were hypothesized to indicate a joy index, and ashamed, embarrassed and humiliated were hypothesized to indicate a shame index. Then, based on factor analyses of the 29 indices, a 3-factor solution for emotions was found: pleasure, arousal and domination. Similarly, Batra and Holbrook (1990) factor analysed 12 emotional indices (largely a subset of those revealed in Holbrook and Batra (1987) with a few exceptions) and discovered 3 factors corresponding closely to those discovered by Edell and Burke (1987). Other researchers (for example Westbrook 1987; Oliver 1994), also using factor analysis, have found emotional items to load on two factors: positive and negative affect.

Richins (1997) has argued that consumption-related emotions are more complex than the two- and three-factor solutions observed in studies of reactions to ads or customer satisfaction. Moreover, because exploratory factor analyses often yield a small number of factors, she utilized a multidimensional scaling procedure, in conjunction with examination of clusters based on location and semantic similarity of emotional descriptors in two-dimensional space. Sixteen clusters of emotions were identified, each measured by between two and eight indicators (in Study 4): anger, discontent, worry, sadness, fear, shame, envy, loneliness, romantic love, love, peacefulness, contentment, optimism, joy, excitement and surprise.

Although the approaches used by consumer researchers to date have been largely empirically driven (for example Edell and Burke 1987; Holbrook and Batra 1987; Westbrook 1987; Oliver 1994; Richins 1997), they are consistent in certain senses with leading perspectives on emotions in psychology. For example, Holbrook and Batra's (1987) three-factor pleasure-arousal-domination findings are similar to Russell and Mehrabian's (1977) three-factor pleasure-arousal-dominance model. However, some differences can be pointed out. The most important are the high loadings of sadness and fear on the domination factor in Holbrook and Batra's (1987) study, in contrast to the more common outcome of sadness loading on or near the negative pole of a pleasure–displeasure factor, and fear loading about 45° away from displeasure and towards greater arousal (for example Russell 1997).

Similarly, the three factors found in Edell and Burke's (1987) study (that is, upbeat feelings, negative feelings and warm feelings), correspond roughly to the high positive affect–low positive affect, high negative affect–low negative affect, and pleasantness–unpleasantness dimensions, respectively, of Watson and Tellegen's (1985) circumplex model; and the positive affect and negative affect factors observed by Oliver (1994) and Westbrook (1987) also align to a great extent with factors on the circumplex model (see also Mano and Oliver 1993).

The circumplex structure of emotions is shown in Figure 3.2. This representation of emotions has also been called the two-factor model, because, based on the techniques used to generate it (for example factor analysis or multidimensional scaling), emotions can be arranged around two orthogonal axes. Russell (1997) terms the axes pleasure–displeasure and arousal–sleepiness, while Watson and Tellegen (1985) label them high positive affect–low positive affect and high negative affect–low negative affect. Russell's interpretation is essentially the same as Watson and Tellegen's pleasantness–unpleasantness and strong engagement–disengagement axes, which are rotated 45° from their primary axes (but see Larsen and Diener 1992).

The idea behind the circumplex model is that emotions exist in bipolar categories (for example happy–sad, nervous–relaxed) and can be arranged in a continuous order around the perimeter of a two-factor space. The closer emotions are to each other on the perimeter, the more similar they are. For example, excited and aroused are more similar than are content and aroused (see Figure 3.2). The origin or centre of the circumplex is thought to represent a neutral point or adaptation level.

The circumplex model is appealing because it is intuitive, simple and provides a description of which emotions are similar and which are dissimilar. However, it has drawbacks. The most serious limitation is that it is based on empirical associations among experienced emotions and has nothing to say about the conditions (for example appraisals) producing emotions. Then, too, the circumplex model can obscure subtle differences in emotions.

Consensual mood structure

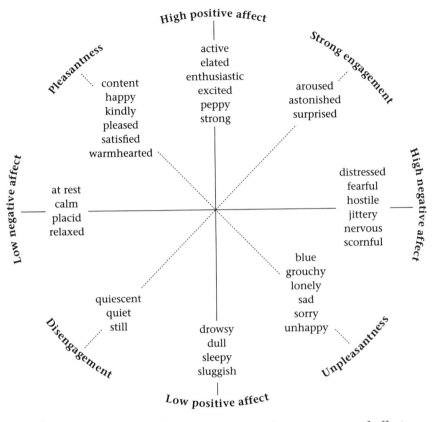

Figure 3.2 Watson and Tellegen's (1985) two-factor structure of affect
Source: Watson and Tellegen (1985: 225). Copyright ©1985 by the American Psychological Association. Reprinted with permission.

Depending on eliciting conditions and people's appraisals, each of the emotions grouped together within any particular category on the circumplex can be distinct from its co-category members. For example, it is possible to feel fearful without feeling hostile (see 'high negative affect' in Figure 3.2). Also the circumplex contains categories that may not correspond to emotions. For instance, surprised, drowsy and sleepy do not seem to reflect emotions. On the other hand, the circumplex fails to represent well instances of emotion important in everyday life and consumption. It does not accommodate love, disgust, pride, hope, guilt, shame or embarrassment very well, to name a few. The various two- and three-factor summaries of emotions disclosed in consumer research also include variables not reflective of emotions and exclude instances generally recognized as emotions.

Richins's (1997) consumption emotions set (CES) with its 16 descriptors is appealing because it covers most emotional reactions one encounters in consumption, and its measures achieved satisfactory reliability (except for measure of envy, loneliness, peacefulness and contentment). The CES would be best used within the context of a particular theory of emotions to operationalization specific categories of emotions hypothesized to serve as antecedents, consequences or moderating variables. The CES could also be used to operationalize emotions in more empirically oriented studies, but whether measures of each dimension would achieve discriminate validity is problematic. Most studies incorporating multiple instances of both positive emotions and negative emotions find that the measures load on two factors corresponding to positive and negative emotions (for example Oliver 1994; Bagozzi et al. 1998).

This raises the question of when one can expect discrete emotional reactions versus amalgamated groupings of, say, positive emotions and negative emotions (for example highly correlated feelings of anger, sadness and fear). The advantage of a theory-based approach to emotions is that specific conditions can be specified for the occurrence of distinct emotions, and these hypotheses can be tested. It is for these reasons that we used appraisal theories as our organizing framework for looking at emotions. Discrete emotional reactions are likely to happen when one manipulates conditions producing specific appraisals or when naturally occurring events correspond to unique appraisal conditions. Gopinath and Bagozzi (2001), for example, were able to induce independent emotional reactions toward three targets in a movie going context. Based on Roseman's (1991) theory, distinct emotional reactions were produced as a function of three-way interactions between motive consistency–inconsistency, appetitive–aversive and self–other agency conditions. For early studies in consumer research where emotions were created through experimental manipulations, see Folkes (1984), Folkes et al. (1987); Taylor (1994); Nyer (1997b).

By contrast, research not based on manipulations of appraisal conditions or based on reactions to a single stimulus frequently finds that emotions cluster in two- and on occasion three-factors (for example Edell and Burke 1987; Holbrook and Batra 1987; Westbrook 1987; Oliver 1994). Further, research examining the construct validity of measures of discrete emotions obtained in non-experimental, survey settings shows that discriminate validity is often lacking among measures of different positive or different negative emotions (for example Bagozzi 1993) or between measures within a particular subcategory of positive or negative emotions, such as among measures of elation, gladness and joy (Bagozzi 1991a).

What accounts for the differences in findings between experimental research based on appraisal theories and survey research or research based on reactions to a single stimulus measured by inventories of emotional items? One possibility may be that discrete emotional reactions are short-lived or, once activated, stimulate other emotional reactions closely related to them.

Consider, for example, sadness: 'when we experience loss, we rarely feel a single emotion such as sadness. We grieve, are angry, anxious, guilty, envious, even hopeful, and defensive' (Lazarus 1991: 250). A reason why these emotions may go in tandem is that coping processes for sadness may involve active struggle or even protest against loss, which results in other emotions. Alternatively, the absence of discrete emotions may simply reflect how difficult it is to create them. As Izard (1972: 103) noted, pure emotions are 'virtually impossible to obtain in the laboratory or in any research setting'. However, as noted above, researchers have recently found that the use of scenarios in an experimental context can generate discrete emotional responses (for example Roseman 1991; Gopinath and Bagozzi 2001).

Another factor that might account for a coalescence of multiple positive emotions and multiple negative emotions in two corresponding groupings is the nature of the stimulus under study. Most stimulus ads, products or brands are complex, and the appraisals engendered are typically variegated, but related. Also the way items are presented on some questionnaires makes it difficult to uncover discrete emotional components. When multiple measures of a single discrete emotional response (for example happy, pleased and joyful for 'joy') are interspersed throughout a questionnaire, this tends to reduce correlations among items purported to indicate the same response and to increase correlations of these items with measures of other responses. The result is predictably a reduction in discriminate validity and high correlations among items measuring positive emotions and among items measuring negative emotions. The alternative is to group items by the emotional response they are intended to tap, which tends to increase correlations among measures of the same thing and decrease correlations among measures of different emotional responses. Thus, a trade-off is entailed by use of either practice.

An issue that has received little attention in consumer research is whether to use unipolar or bipolar items to measure emotions. The choice can influence findings and their interpretation in fundamental ways. Some leading scholars claim that emotions are in the final analysis bipolar states or processes. We are either happy or sad, for example, and any other pattern (for example independence or concomitance) is thought to be an artifact of measurement error. Although a number of studies have shown that pleasant and unpleasant emotions are independent (for example Bradburn 1969; Zevon and Tellegen 1982; Diener and Emmons 1985), D.P. Green et al. (1993) and Barrett and Russell (1998) argue and present findings demonstrating that emotions are bipolar, once random or both random and systematic errors are taken into account (see also Russell and Carroll 1999).

Bagozzi et al. (1999b) challenge the conclusions made by D.P. Green et al. (1993) and Barrett and Russell (1998). They hypothesize that bipolarity, independence and concomitance depend on gender, culture, and the target of one's emotions. Briefly, Bagozzi et al. (1999b) found that positive and negative emotions were highly negatively correlated for American women but highly positively correlated for Chinese women. The former pattern is evidence for bipolarity (that is, either positive or negative emotions occur but not both), the latter for concomitance (that is, both positive and negative emotions occur at the same time). For men, the correlations between positive and negative emotions were much smaller in magnitude but in the same direction across ethnicity: that is, slight negative correlations were found for American men, slight positive correlations for Chinese men. Thus, the relationship between positive and negative emotions for men was nearly independent. Bagozzi et al. (1999b) argued that differences in culture (that is, a tendency for Americans to view things in dichotomies or discrete categories, in opposition; and a tendency for Chinese to view things dialectically, that is, in balance or harmony) interact with gender differences (that is, a tendency for women to be more knowledgeable about and skilled in the use of emotions than men) to produce the divergent patterns. The above findings resulted when people were asked to express how they felt at the moment according to their idiosyncratic reasons, which is the standard procedure used in the literature. That is, the stimulus for each person could be considered heterogeneous across subjects. However, when Americans and Chinese were asked to give their emotional reactions to eating in fast food restaurants (a common, singular stimulus), positive and negative emotions were independent for men and women alike (not presented in Bagozzi et al. 1999b).

It is perhaps too early to give definitive recommendations on which emotional scales to employ in empirical work, but for now, we think that it is advisable to use unipolar scales that ask respondents to express to what extent each emotion describes their own subjective feelings, rather than bipolar scales which can obscure differences in emotional responses across the various dimensions. Also, at least five, preferably seven to nine, scale steps should be used for each item to enhance the chances that optimal distributional properties of measures will be achieved. In addition, at least three, preferably more, items should be used for each emotional subcategory.

A final measurement issue we wish to raise is the following. To what extent are emotions blends of categories? For ease of discussion, we consider the categories of emotions presented on the circumplex. Pleasantness–unpleasantness might combine, for instance, with arousal to produce different kinds or intensities of emotion. To take a particular example, consider happiness, an instance of pleasantness on the circumplex. Intense forms of happiness occur when pleasantness combines with high arousal: elated, excited, enthusiastic, euphoric, gleeful, joyous, ecstatic and exultant are examples. Mild forms of happiness occur when pleasantness combines with low arousal: peaceful, calm, serene or quietude of mind are examples. Everyday happiness might be at an intermediate level of arousal. For other views on happiness, see Bagozzi (1999). Other perspectives on blended emotions, based not on a blend of arousal with emotion categories but rather on combinations of 'basic' emotions, can be found in Izard (1991, 1992) and Plutchik (1980).

What more general role, if any, does arousal play in emotions (Bagozzi 1991b)? We turn to this issue next.

Arousal

An early, influential point of view on emotions was professed by James (1890: 449) who claimed that *'bodily changes follow directly the perception of the exciting fact, and . . . our feeling of the same changes as they occur IS the emotion'* (emphasis in original). For James, different stimuli lead to different bodily responses (for example sweaty palms, racing heart, and so on), these physiological responses are then detected as bodily sensations in our mind, and the result is interpreted by us as emotional experiences. But it is important to note that James reserved this interpretation for what he termed the 'coarser' emotions (for example 'grief, fear, rage, love') which involve strong bodily perturbations; he was less clear about what he termed the 'subtler' emotions (for example 'moral, intellectual, and aesthetic feelings': James 1890: 468).

An equally influential theory of emotions was proposed by Schachter and Singer (1962) who argued that emotion is essentially bodily arousal plus a cognitive label one provides to diagnose one's felt arousal, a perspective consistent with James's point of view. The idea is that we first experience physiological arousal, and, especially when we are unaware or uncertain of the origin of the arousal, we look for evidence in the physical and social situation accompanying the arousal to label our emotional state. Although this theory had considerable impact in psychology for nearly three decades, it has largely been discredited and has not received much supporting evidence beyond Schachter and Singer's (1962) original experiment (for example Manstead and Wagner 1981; Reisenzein 1983). One exception to the above observation is the frequently repeated finding that arousal misattributed to an extraneous source intensifies emotions (for example Zillman 1971; Cantor et al. 1974; Dutton and Aron 1974).

An important contribution of James (1890) and Schachter and Singer (1962) was the recognition that arousal plays an essential role in emotion. Before we address arousal more fully, we should mention studies in consumer research that address the acquisition of affect, without necessarily involving concepts of arousal or information processing. Considerable emphasis has been placed on the effects of various stimuli on consumer behaviour. Retail store environment cues, advertising, background music, brand names, packages, celebrity endorsers and other stimuli are frequently administered to produce emotional reactions in consumers. The premise is that emotions or moods trigger buying responses (for example Gardner 1985; Hill and Gardner 1987).

If not by appraisal processes or direct arousal, per se, how does presentation of a stimulus under repetitive conditions induce affect? A seductively simple explanation was provided by Zajonc who argued that 'when objects are presented to the individual on repeated occasions, the mere exposure is capable of making the individual's attitude toward these objects more posit- ive' (Zajonc and Markus 1982: 125). This 'mere exposure' effect has been found primarily when the stimulus is simple and previously unknown or else has little or no semantic content (for example nonsense syllables, foreign words). One mechanism that has been offered to explain the **mere exposure effect** is familiarity: we come to like things that are familiar to us, perhaps because of feelings of security (Zajonc 1968). However, a full theoretical explanation for the mere exposure effect has not been developed. When a person is exposed to meaningful stimuli, it has been more difficult to produce the mere exposure effect (for example Obermiller 1985). This is, in part, a consequence of the cognitive processing that occurs in response to awareness of the meaningful stimuli. Repeated exposure to a meaningful stimulus can lead to increased or decreased positive or negative feelings, depending on its meaning. Mere exposure, thus, loses its utility in such cases, both as a theory and a practical tactic.

Based loosely on the notion that emotions or moods induced by one stimulus become attached to another, some researchers have investigated the effects of (a) music on length of stay and money spent in supermarkets and restaurants (for example Milliman 1982, 1986) and (b) affective tone of stores on purchase intentions (for example Donovan and Rossiter 1982) and evaluations (for example Gardner and Simokos 1986). How can the observed attachment of affect from one stimulus to another be explained? Shimp (1991) reviews seven studies in consumer research that test various facets of classical conditioning explanations. The idea behind classical conditioning is that the repeated pairing of a conditioned stimulus (for example a new brand name) with an unconditioned stimulus (for example an attractive spokesperson) will eventually lead to the new brand name, on its own, stimulating the unconditioned response (for example positive affect) origin- ally induced by the unconditioned stimulus. Very few studies have been performed in consumer research that conform to the conditions required to test classical conditioning. It is unclear whether classical conditioning studies can be designed to rule out such rival explanations as demand char- acteristics or cognitive interpretations of the results. Allen and Janiszewski (1989) provide some evidence that at least one type of cognitive mediation is necessary for classical conditioning to occur: namely, awareness of the contingency between the conditioned stimulus and unconditioned stimulus. On the other hand, classical conditioning, particularly for fear responses, has been shown to involve unconscious arousal processes connected with the amygdala (LeDoux 1996).

Another way to explain the observed attachment of affect from one stimu- lus to another is by Zillman's (1971) excitation-transfer model. Briefly, Zillman proposed that exposure to one stimulus may produce arousal. If a second stimulus is presented close on that also is capable of producing arousal on its own, the two sources of arousal may combine to produce intensely experi- enced arousal. Under certain conditions (for example unawareness of the source of arousal from the first stimulus, recency of the second), a person may attribute the arousal to the second stimulus. Zillman (1983) interpreted arousal as undifferentiated sympathetic activation.

An issue in need of resolution is whether emotions can occur without arousal. Cognitive theories of emotions (for example appraisal theories) seem to allow that emotions can be produced by cognition alone, without arousal (for example Parrott 1988). But does arousal always accompany the experience of emotions?

Research suggests that arousal is an essential component of emotion and is manifest in neural systems in the brain. LeDoux (1996) reviews evidence suggesting that there are at least five arousal systems in the brain contributing complexly to emotional experience. Four of these are in regions of the brain stem and rely respectively on acetylcholine, noradrenaline, dopamine, and serotonin for activation. A fifth (the nucleus basalis) is in the forebrain and also relies on acetylcholine to arouse cortical cells. LeDoux (1996) notes that the arousal systems act in nonspecific ways throughout the forebrain to make cells more sensitive to incoming signals. In a sense, the nonspecific arousal interacts with the information processing of a particular stimulus. The amygdala acts as a kind of central processor and interacts with the prefrontal cortex (working memory and attention), hippocampus (long-term explicit memory) and sensory cortex (perception and short-term storage) to influence emotional responses. The amygdala not only influences cortical areas of the brain, but also receives input from arousal networks (which themselves also influence the forebrain) and feedback from bodily expression of emotions. In addition, signals from the amygdala are sent to muscles and internal organs and glands.

Most of the research to date into the role of arousal systems and the amygdala in emotional behavior has been limited to a small number of emotions (for example fear). But it is believed that each emotional response is mediated by separate neural systems, although each may overlap or resemble each other in many respects. In sum, LeDoux (1996) and other brain researchers (for example Damasio 1994) construe emotions as biological functions of the nervous system (see also Zajonc 1998).

To our knowledge, there has been little work to either integrate or reconcile cognitive theories of emotions with neural and biological theories. Much remains to be done in psychological research before we can make definitive statements about the precise role of arousal in emotional experience and behaviour.

At least three studies have examined limited aspects of arousal in consumption contexts. Sanbonmatsu and Kardes (1988) found that arousal may govern attitude formation in persuasive message settings. Attitudes were based on peripheral cues, when subjects were highly aroused, but on argument strength when they were moderately aroused. It is unclear whether arousal functioned here to reduce information processing capacity of external arguments or focused attention on internal reactions.

Bagozzi (1994b) found that, consistent with predictions by knowledge-assembly theory (Hayes-Roth 1977), arousal transformed a two-dimensional, affective-cognitive representation of evaluations of giving blood into a one-dimensional, unitized representation. Likewise, arousal increased the association between attitudes and positive beliefs about the consequences of giving blood and decreased the association between attitudes and negative beliefs. These predictions on the associations between attitudes and beliefs were explained by the implications of spreading activation effects of arousal and coping responses, wherein subjects attempt to avoid negative and facilitate positive associations of beliefs with attitudes. In another study, Bagozzi (1996) found that, for attitudes toward giving blood, high arousal tends to enhance a halo effect from attitudes to positive beliefs and reduce the halo from attitudes to negative beliefs about the consequences of giving blood.

Clearly, arousal is a fundamental aspect of behaviour related to emotions. We must acknowledge that appraisal theories have not done a good, or at least complete, job of incorporating arousal into their frameworks. In their defence, however, we should mention the following. Appraisal theorists recognize that the intensity of emotional experience consists of two components: arousal and self-control (for example Frijda 1994: 120). Likewise, researchers accept that 'autonomic nervous system and other physiological processes' at least accompany subjectively felt emotions (for example Oatley 1992: 21) and that '[i]f the criterion of physiological activity was eliminated from the definition, the concept of emotion would be left without one of the important response boundaries with which to distinguish it from nonemotion' (Lazarus 1991: 58–9). But is there more to arousal in emotion than this?

Some psychologists and marketers have been quick to dismiss Zajonc's claim that 'preferences need no inferences' (Zajonc 1980; see Lazarus 1982; Marcel 1983; Zajonc 1984; Cohen and Areni 1991: 215–16). However, we believe it is important, at the present, to recognize that emotional meanings can be processed subconsciously, emotions can be activated automatically, and responses to emotions (for example coping, action tendencies, actions) also can occur automatically. We leave open the possibility that 'emotion and cognition are best thought of as separate but interacting mental functions mediated by separate but interacting brain systems' (LeDoux 1996: 69; see also Oatley 1992: ch. 1). It appears that arousal is a key part of emotional functions in the brain that underlies much of its automaticity. Cognitive appraisals and arousal need to be better incorporated into our theories of emotion.

Emotions as markers, mediators and moderators of consumer responses

Based on content, most advertisements can be divided into two categories: (a) thinking ads, where focus is placed on either factual information (for example product attributes) or utilitarian consequences of product/service usage (for example savings in time or money) or (b) feeling ads, where concentration is placed on the emotions one will experience through use or ownership of a product (see Puto and Wells's (1984), similar distinction between informational and transformational advertising). Rather than focusing on the stimulus, per se, it is more important to emphasize the processes and experiences comprising a consumer's response to ads, in order to better understand the emotional meaning of ads (for example Friestad and Thorson 1986).

Paralleling the above differentiation between types of ads and the emotional-cognitive division in mental processes mentioned earlier, Batra and Ray (1986) developed a framework and coding scheme for classifying affective responses to ads, as a complement to **cognitive responses**. Specifically, Batra and Ray (1986) identified three positive affective response categories: surgency-elation-vigour/activation (SEVA), deactivation, and social affection feelings. The SEVA feelings refer to upbeat, happy mood reactions (for example 'the ad's music was "catchy", the ad was "fun to watch or breezy", or . . . a likable use of humor'), deactivation includes soothing, relaxing, quiet or pleasing reactions, and social affection encompasses feelings of warmth, tenderness and caring (Batra and Ray 1986: 241). The three positive affective responses were used along with six cognitive responses (that is, support arguments, counter arguments, execution discounting, execution bolstering, neutral distracters and other reactions) in a study of the impact of television commercials on consumers. A total of 12 per cent of reactions to ads were classified as positive affect: SEVA (3.7 per cent), deactivation (2.5 per cent) and social affect (6.1 per cent).

One use of emotional reactions in the above sense might be as markers or indicators of the effectiveness of advertising copy, particularly with respect to the overall persuasiveness of the ad, the appeal of spokespersons, evaluation of particular product claims, and appraisals of other aspects of the execution (Wiles and Cornwell 1990). Also the programme surrounding an ad (for example happy versus sad content) has been found to have main effects on one's evaluation of an ad and recall (for example Goldberg and Gorn 1987). Future research is needed to identify how programme content and advertising appeals interact to influence consumer emotional responses.

A research question that has received quite a bit of attention in recent years is how, and to what extent, do emotional reactions to ads influence consumer decision making. Most often these reactions have been measured as attitudes (for example liking) toward the ad (for example Mitchell and Olson 1981; Shimp 1981; Brown and Stayman 1992).

Attitude toward the ad (A_{ad}) is thought to be a function of feelings (and thoughts) about the ad itself (for example Batra and Ray 1986; Mackenzie et al. 1986). In fact, Batra and Ray (1986) found that the three affective responses discussed above significantly predicted A_{ad} even after controlling for the effects of cognitive responses. A number of researchers have examined the conditions under which emotions influence A_{ad}. For instance, under low involvement viewing conditions, feelings about the ad have been found to be more important determinants of A_{ad} than thoughts (for example how informative or useful the ad is), but under higher involvement viewing, both feelings and thoughts may be important (for example Miniard et al. 1990). Presumably, high involvement promotes cognitive processing of the usefulness of the ad and its content.

A majority of research has addressed the effects of A_{ad}, especially on attitudes toward the brand (A_b). Classic attitude theory maintains that A_b is a function of beliefs about brand attributes or consequences of product use. Mitchell and Olson (1981) and Shimp (1981) were the first to find that A_{ad} provided additional explanatory power for A_b over and above brand beliefs (see also Edell and Burke 1987). Batra and Ray (1986) found, however, that affective responses towards the ad influenced A_b only indirectly through A_{ad}.

Some research has addressed the conditions under which A_{ad} influences A_b. For example, Brown and Stayman (1992) revealed in their meta-analysis that the effects of A_{ad} on A_b are greater for novel than well-known brands and for durable and other goods versus non-durables. Some evidence also exists showing that A_{ad} influences A_b indirectly through its effect on beliefs about the brand (Mackenzie et al. 1986). Finally, Stayman and Aaker (1988) showed that repetition governs the feelings to A_{ad} relationship. Under levels of low versus high repetition, feelings have a stronger effect on A_{ad}. This may be a consequence of greater information processing under high versus low repetition.

In addition to the transfer of affect from ad emotions to A_{ad}, research shows that brand names and feelings towards ads can become linked in memory. Stayman and Batra (1991) found that subjects exposed to an affective, as opposed to an argument, ad were able to retrieve brand attitudes faster, when primed with the brand name. In addition, the positive retrieved affect had a stronger influence on choice in low than in high involvement contexts. In a second study, Stayman and Batra (1991) demonstrated that viewers of an ad who were in a positive affective state more strongly evoked the affect when given the brand name as a subsequent retrieval cue than viewers exposed to the ad while not in a positive affect state.

Olney et al. (1991) investigated a hierarchical model explaining advertising viewing time. The effects of ad emotions (that is, pleasure and arousal) were mediated by A_{ad} and reactions to ad content. Interestingly, arousal had both indirect and direct effects on viewing time, even after controlling for ad content and A_{ad}. Arousal was measured by self-reports.

Emotions have been found to serve as moderators in their impact on A_b. Batra and Stayman (1990), in one of the few studies to examine mood and print ads, found that positive moods enhance A_b through their interaction with two cognitive processes: '(1) a bias against the generation of negative thoughts (such as evoked by weak arguments), leading to a more favourable evaluation of message arguments, and (2) a reduction in total cognitive elaboration, making processing more heuristic than systematic' (Batra and Stayman 1990: 212–13). An interesting finding was that positive moods seem to reduce counter-argumentation when weak arguments are used in ads (see also Worth and Mackie 1987). Batra and Stephens (1994) also investigated the moderating effects of mood on A_b. Specifically, they showed that mood and motivation (the latter conceived as degree of relevance of the product category for consumers) interacted to govern A_b, when consumers watched television ads. The greatest impact on A_b occurred when positive moods ensued under conditions of low motivation. The rationale is that positive moods and low motivation suppress counter-argumentation (and therefore lead to more favourable A_b) in comparison to high motivation conditions.

The effects of emotion on cognitive processes

A person's emotional state can influence various aspects of information processing including encoding and retrieval of information, different strategies used to process information, evaluations and judgements, and creative thinking.

Emotion/mood effects on memory

The influence of mood states on memory can be broadly classified into three categories: retrieval effects, encoding effects and state-dependent learning effects.

Retrieval effects
Affect has been shown to influence retrieval of information, whereby persons in a positive mood state at the time of retrieval have been found to show superior recall of positive material learned during encoding, relative to neutral or negative material (Isen et al. 1978; Laird et al. 1982; Nasby and Yando 1982; Teasdale and Russell 1983). For example, Isen et al. (1978) had subjects study positive, negative and neutral words. Either positive, neutral or negative mood states were induced in these subjects. Subjects in the positive mood condition retrieved more positive words compared to neutral or negative words. Isen et al. (1978) suggest that thinking about mood incongruent material involves shifting one's focus, which is cognitively taxing, and therefore people are more likely to focus on mood congruent material. Another mechanism proposed to explain the retrieval effects of positive affect suggests that positive mood at the time of retrieval functions as a cue that primes the positive material in memory, making these material more accessible (Isen et al. 1978; Isen 1989; see also Tulving and Pearlstone 1966 for a discussion on the effects of priming on **accessibility**). The easier accessibility of positive material may then influence other cognitive processes such as evaluations and decision making, and also subsequent behaviours. While

retrieval effects have been replicated by many researchers using different mood induction and testing techniques, a few prominent studies have failed to detect retrieval effects (Bower et al. 1978; Bower et al. 1981), leading Isen (1984) to speculate that this failure may have been caused by the specific material and induction methods (such as hypnosis) used in these studies.

Encoding effects

Mood states have also been shown to exhibit encoding effects whereby the affective state at the time of learning is associated with superior memory for similarly valenced material (Bower and Cohen 1982; Forgas and Bower 1987). Nasby and Yando (1982) found that positive mood at the time of learning led to an improved recall of positive material at a later point in time regardless of the mood state at the time of recall. Bower et al. (1981) found evidence for the encoding effect of both positive and negative affect. Subjects were made to feel happy or sad and then read descriptions of various psychiatric interviews. Happy subjects learned many more happy facts than sad facts, while sad subjects learned many more sad facts than happy facts.

How can the encoding effects of mood be explained? Bower and Cohen (1982) suggested that mood congruent material is likely to be more semantically elaborated relative to mood incongruent material. Forgas and Bower (1987) found that in impression formation situations, sad subjects spent more time examining negative rather than positive information, and subsequently recalled the negative information better. Conversely, happy subjects spent more time on the positive information and recalled that better at a later time. The greater levels of associations evoked by mood congruent material may have caused more extensive elaboration, which in turn requires more time. However, Isen et al. (1978) and Srull (1983) failed to find any encoding effects of affect.

State-dependent learning effects

A third memory effect of mood is the state-dependent learning effect of affect, where any material regardless of its affective valence learned under a particular mood state is recalled better when the person is again in that affective state (Bower et al. 1978; Bartlett and Santrock 1979; Bower et al. 1981; Bartlett et al. 1982). Bower et al. (1978) had subjects learn two sets of words, one while they were in a positive affective state and the other in a negative mood. When subjects who learned the two lists in different moods recalled the words in the wrong mood (for example when words learned in a positive mood were recalled while subjects were in a negative mood), they experienced interference and the average recall rate was less than 50 per cent. When subjects who learned two lists in different moods recalled the words in the correct mood, the average recall rate was over 70 per cent. Control subjects who learned and recalled both lists while in the same mood showed an average recall rate between 50 and 60 per cent. Bower and Cohen (1982) suggest that the subject's mood at the time of learning becomes associated with the learned material, and that these associations facilitate the recall of learned material when the mood state at recall matches the mood state at encoding (see also Bower 1981).

Evidence for mood state-dependent learning has been ambiguous. Many studies have failed to find any state-dependent effects of mood-state (Isen et al. 1978; Laird et al. 1982; Nasby and Yando 1982; Bower and Mayer 1985). Eich and Birnbaum (1982) and Isen (1984, 1989) have suggested that when the material to be learned has semantic meaning, the stimulus will be encoded according to this meaning, and the influence of the mood state in the encoding and subsequent retrieval processes will be minimal. However, when the stimulus lacks meaning, contextual cues such as affective states at the time of learning may be more strongly encoded with the learned material. At the time of retrieval, these memory items, which have few semantic associations, are more primed by the matching affective state at recall.

Asymmetric effects of positive and negative moods
While positive affective states have been shown to have significant influences on recall, negative affect has sometimes been found to have either no effect, or a much smaller effect on the recall of negative material from memory. Asymmetric effects of positive and negative moods have been found for retrieval effects (Isen et al. 1978; Teasdale and Fogarty 1979; Nasby and Yando 1982), encoding effects (Nasby and Yando 1982) and state-dependent learning effects (Bartlett and Santrock 1979; Bartlett et al. 1982). Isen (1984) speculated that positive affect is structured in a broad and extensive manner (that is, highly interconnected with other memories), while negative affect is more narrowly and less well connected with other material, and that specific negative affective states such as anger and sadness may be organized separately in memory. This, in turn, would make it difficult for any given negative mood to act as an effective retrieval cue. It is not readily apparent why negative affect would be less well connected in memory and positive affect more widely interconnected as Isen suggests, considering that negative affect usually signals problematic environmental conditions that may require problem solving (Schwarz and Clore 1983; Wegener et al. 1995). One of the side-effects of this hypothesized interconnectedness of positive memories is the greater creativeness and cognitive flexibility demonstrated by people in positive moods.

Mood maintenance and repair have also been put forward as explanations for the asymmetric effects of positive and negative moods. Isen (1984) has suggested that happy subjects attempt to prolong their positive affective state by focusing on the positive aspects of their stimulus (mood maintenance), while subjects in a negative mood try to improve their situation by not focusing on negative memories (mood repair). Isen (1989) noted that in some of the studies showing symmetrical effects of positive and negative mood (Bower et al. 1978, 1981), subjects were instructed to maintain their induced moods, and this may have discouraged them from engaging in mood repair strategies. However, the mood repair explanation is not without problems. If sad subjects engage in mood repair, why is there no evidence for mood incongruent recall effects? After all, an effective strategy to improve a depressed mood state is to engage in pleasant thoughts and memories. Yet, evidence seems to show that negative mood inhibits the recall of positive memories (Isen et al. 1978). The competing explanations of memory structure differences and mood maintenance/repair have also been used to explain differences in information processing strategies of happy and sad individuals.

Mood, categorization and creativity

Studies have found that people in positive mood states, compared to those in neutral or negative mood states, tend to be better at integrating information, finding relationships among stimuli and at finding creative solutions (Isen and Daubman 1984; Isen et al. 1985, 1987; Murray et al. 1990; Isen et al. 1992). For example, subjects in positive mood conditions tended to group a wider range of neutral stimuli together (Isen and Daubman 1984). They also rated words such as *cane*, *ring* and *purse* as being better exemplars of the category 'clothing', than did the neutral mood subjects. Murray et al. (1990) found that positive mood subjects, compared to subjects in other mood states, formed broader categories when focusing on similarities among exemplars, and narrower categories when focusing on differences, prompting them to suggest that what positive mood promotes is not broader categorization, but rather cognitive flexibility. Isen et al. (1985) found that positive mood subjects tended to give more unusual responses to neutral words in word association tests. For example in response to the word 'house', positive mood subjects were more likely than neutral mood subjects to mention unusual first associates such as *security*, *residence* and *apartment*, suggesting that positive mood states may influence cognitive organization, resulting in more flexible interpretation of relationships among stimuli. This cognitive flexibility also results in enhanced creativity. Isen et al. (1987) found that subjects in positive mood states outperformed those in neutral and negative mood states on tests requiring creative solutions. These researchers suggest that positive mood subjects were better at creative problem solving since such tasks require the ability to see relatedness among seemingly unrelated stimuli, and as we have seen earlier, positive affect results in more flexible cognitive organization.

Mood effects on evaluation

One of the best recognized and most robust effects of mood is its influence on evaluation. Individuals in positive mood states have been shown to evaluate stimuli more positively than individuals in neutral or negative mood states, whether the stimuli being studied are other people (Clore and Byrne 1974; Forgas and Bower 1987), consumer goods (Isen et al. 1978; Srull 1983), life satisfaction (Schwarz and Clore 1983), or past life events (Clark and Teasdale 1982). The reliability of mood effects on evaluation is perhaps best illustrated by the fact that evaluations of the pleasantness of neutral/ambiguous stimuli are used as checks for mood manipulation (for example Isen et al. 1985, 1987). Isen et al. (1978) found that subjects in whom positive mood was induced were more likely to rate their cars and televisions more favourably compared to subjects in neutral mood states. In the case of memory based evaluations, if the recalled information is biased by the mood, then evaluations that follow will be biased too. Online processing of evaluations can also be influenced by mood states through the retrieval of information congruent with the mood (Clore et al. 1994).

A competing explanation based on the feelings-as-information model (see Schwarz 1990; Schwarz and Clore 1983; Schwarz and Bless 1991) suggests that subjects may assume that their mood states are affective reactions to the object being evaluated, and thus base their evaluations on their affective states. For example, a happy individual when asked to evaluate a painting, may ask the question 'How do I feel?' and infer that their positive mood is a reaction to the painting, and therefore come to the conclusion that they like the painting. The feelings-as-information hypothesis suggests that when subjects attribute their mood state to something else other than the object being evaluated, the effect of mood on evaluation should disappear. Schwarz and Clore (1983) found support for this hypothesis when they showed that, although people called on sunny days reported more life satisfaction than people called on cloudy days, the differences disappeared when the interviewer casually mentioned the weather to the subjects. Presumably, the mention of the weather made people attribute their mood to the weather, and hence the mood lost any diagnostic value in evaluating life satisfaction. In other words, people may use their moods as the basis for forming evaluations of objects unless the diagnostic value of the mood is discounted. Clore et al. (1994) compared the two explanations for mood effects on evaluation and suggested that individuals may use feelings as information when the evaluation task is affective in nature, when other information is lacking, when the information is complex, or when there are time constraints.

Although mood effects on evaluation have been replicated often, a few prominent studies have shown that mood states do not influence evaluation when the object being evaluated is highly familiar and for which past evaluations exist in memory (for example Srull 1983, 1984; Salovey and Birnbaum 1989). Srull (1984: experiment 3) found that the evaluations of a car made by novices, but not by experts, were influenced by mood state. Novices, by definition, are unfamiliar with the product category, and are more likely to engage in online evaluations, which are more susceptible to mood influences. Experts, on the other hand, have prior evaluations available in memory, and so do not engage in online evaluations and are less likely to be influenced by mood. Similar findings have been obtained by Salovey and Birnbaum (1989: experiment 3) and Schwarz et al. (1987).

Mood effects on information processing

It has been suggested that the mood maintenance strategy used by people in positive moods may also cause them to avoid investing cognitive effort in tasks unless doing so promises to maintain or enhance their positive mood (for example Isen 1987; Wegener et al. 1995). Consequently, people in positive mood states may not be motivated to engage in systematic processing of information, and may use heuristic processing instead. Positive affect usually denotes a benign environment that does not require any action. On the other hand, negative affective states act as information signalling that the environment poses a problem and may motivate people to engage in systematic processing, which is usually better suited to handling threatening situations (Schwarz and Clore 1983; Schwarz 1990). Various studies have found evidence suggesting the use of heuristic processing by people in positive moods, and systematic processing by people in negative moods (for example Mackie and Worth 1989; Bless et al. 1990, 1996). Bless et al. (1990) presented happy and sad subjects with either strong or weak counter-attitudinal arguments. Sad subjects were influenced only by strong arguments, while happy subjects were equally influenced by strong and weak arguments. These effects have been consistently replicated and have been interpreted as providing evidence for reduced systematic processing by subjects in positive affective states. The two major mechanisms that have been used to explain mood effects on information processing strategies are the same as those used to explain the asymmetric effects of mood effects on memory: namely, the highly interconnected nature of positive memories and mood maintenance.

In discussing the asymmetric effects of positive and negative affect on memory, we had briefly discussed Isen's (1984) contention that positive concepts are more highly interconnected in memory relative to negative ideas. Isen (1987) and Mackie and Worth (1989) have argued that, since positive memories are highly interconnected, positive mood will prime and activate some related and many unrelated positive memories, thus leading to cognitive capacity constraints. Since individuals do not have the cognitive resources to engage in systematic processing, they resort to the less demanding heuristic processing.

A second explanation for mood effects on cognitive processing is based on the concept of mood maintenance. Isen (1987) has suggested that individuals in a positive affective state are motivated to maintain their mood and may avoid cognitive activity that could interfere with their positive mood. Thus, subjects in a happy mood are unlikely to engage in systematic processing of information (also see Bohner et al. 1992).

Another motivation-based explanation for the reduced processing under positive mood has been offered by Schwarz and colleagues (for example Schwarz and Clore 1983) using their feelings-as-information hypothesis. Negative affective states inform people that they may be facing a problem and this may provoke systematic processing of information which is better suited to problem solving. Positive mood, on the other hand, informs the individual that the environment is benign and thus the individual may not be motivated to engage in effortful cognitive processing. A fourth hypothesis suggests that the motivation to simplify processing is not what causes the reliance on heuristic processing, but rather it is the increased use of heuristic processing by these happy mood individuals that results in simplified processing (for example Bless et al. 1996).

Forgas (1994, 1995), building upon Fiedler's (1990) dual-force model, has presented the *affect infusion model* which suggests that the various explanations for mood effects on memory and information processing (such as mood maintenance, feelings-as-information, affect priming) are not necessarily competing models but could rather be, complementary explanations. He suggests that affect infusion into judgemental processes takes place when the judgements require a high degree of constructive (online) processing. Affect does not influence those judgements that call for the retrieval of pre-existing evaluations, or for information processing that is highly specific and not requiring constructive processing. Forgas (1994, 1995) suggests that *direct access processing* (a low affect infusion strategy) is used when the evaluative target is familiar and when there are no strong cognitive, affective, or situational factors that call for systematic processing. Accordingly, individuals who evaluate very familiar objects would be using direct access processing, and hence mood effects would not be found in such cases (cf. Srull 1984). Another low affect infusion strategy is *motivated processing*, where the information search and the evaluative outcome are guided by prior motivational goals such as mood repair (see Forgas 1995 for a detailed discussion). When the evaluative target is simple, the personal relevance is low, the individual has limited cognitive capacity, or the accuracy requirements are not high, the individual may resort to *heuristic processing*, a high affect infusion strategy. Under these circumstances, evaluations may be based on the existing mood, as in the feelings-as-information hypothesis (cf. Schwarz and Bless 1991). When the judgemental situation requires the individual to learn and process novel information, and when he or she has adequate cognitive capacity and motivation to process the information, *substantive processing* is predicted to take place. According to Forgas (1995), this default strategy, which is used if other less effortful strategies are inadequate, involves constructive processing and is one that is susceptible to affect infusion (cf. Srull 1984).

Emotions and customer satisfaction

Early research viewed customer satisfaction as a key outcome of product/ service purchase, whereby a comparison is made between expectations of performance and actual performance, and satisfaction arises when actual performance is greater than or equal to expected performance, and dissatisfaction occurs otherwise (for example Oliver 1980; Yi 1990a). Westbrook (1987) explored the influence of positive affect and negative affect on satisfaction, along with expectation beliefs and disconfirmation beliefs. Satisfaction with automobiles was a function of positive affect, negative affect, expectations of receiving benefits and liabilities, and disconfirmation beliefs. Satisfaction with cable television was determined by positive affect, negative affect, and disconfirmation beliefs. Westbrook and Oliver (1991) found that three emotional responses were important antecedents of satisfaction of newly purchased automobiles: pleasant surprise, interest and hostility.

Oliver (1993) expanded the determinants of satisfaction to include positive affect (interest and joy) and negative affect (anger, disgust, contempt, shame, guilt, fear, sadness), as well as disconfirmation beliefs. In addition, attribute satisfactions and attribute dissatisfactions were hypothesized as direct determinants of satisfaction, as well as indirect (through positive and negative affect) determinants. Satisfaction with automobiles was found to be a function of attribute satisfaction, attribute dissatisfaction, positive affect, negative affect and disconfirmation. Satisfaction with a required university course was also found to be determined by these antecedents, except attribute dissatisfaction.

The investigation of the impact of emotions on post purchase reactions is an important development in consumer research. However, it is unclear whether satisfaction is phenomenologically distinct from many other positive emotions. Satisfaction is neither a basic emotion nor a central emotional category in leading theories of emotions (for example Smith and Ellsworth 1985; Frijda 1986; Lazarus 1991; Roseman 1991; Oatley 1992). Further, Shaver et al. (1987) found that satisfaction shares much common variance with such positive emotions as happiness, joy, gladness, elation, delight and enjoyment, among others. Likewise, Nyer (1997a) discovered that measures of joy and satisfaction loaded on one factor.

Although we leave open the possibility that measures of satisfaction can achieve discriminant validity from measures of joy, happiness and other positive emotions, we believe that this will be very difficult to produce in practice. Also, no theory exists for specifying the conditions under which satisfaction exists uniquely from many other positive emotions. We suspect that previous studies finding discriminant validity for measures of satisfaction can be explained by the way items were presented on the questionnaire (for example separation of measures of satisfaction from measures of other positive emotions) or the lack of inclusion of a sufficient number of positive emotions. No study to date has performed either a rigorous experimental or survey (for example multitrait-multimethod) examination of construct validity of measures of satisfaction, joy and related positive emotions.

The centrality of satisfaction in consumer research is perhaps more due to being the first emotion to receive scrutiny in post-purchase behaviour research than to constituting a unique, fundamental construct in and of itself. Indeed, it is likely that – depending on the situation, product and person – other positive and negative emotions are more important outcomes of purchase. Under certain conditions, frustration, anger, disappointment, alienation, disgust, anxiety, alarm, guilt, shame, joy, happiness, hope, pride, jubilation, excitement, relief, amusement and pleasure, among many other negative and positive emotions, might be more valid reactions that consumers have to purchases. By the same token, the implications of emotional reactions in purchase situations on complaint behaviours, word of mouth communication, repurchase and related actions may differ for various positive and negative emotions and be of more relevance than reactions to satisfaction or dissatisfaction, per se.

Research by Nyer (1997a, 1997b) addresses appraisal theories and their role in post-consumption responses. Nyer found that such post-consumption responses as repurchase intentions, word of mouth intentions, and other reactions are predicted best by using measures of satisfaction plus measures of other emotions. Other studies of note investigating the role of specific emotions in customer satisfaction include those done by Folkes et al. (1987), Taylor (1994) and Dubé et al. (1996).

Some researchers have shifted research from satisfaction, per se, to customer loyalty issues. For example, Smith and Bolton (1998) and Smith et al. (1999) have examined failure and recovery in service contexts. Customer complaints and marketer responses are also important in service contexts (Tax and Chandrashekaran 1998). Some research suggests that repeated experience with a brand or service or loyalty may inoculate or build resistance in consumers to product/service failures or negative publicity (and perhaps even product/service improvements) under some conditions (Ahluwalia et al. 2000). Pre-existing attitudes or **attitude accessibility** may play a role here (Allen et al. 1992; Fazio et al. 2000).

We are uncertain whether a single, summary emotional response such as 'satisfaction' is feasible or even desirable. But if one is to be discovered, it may lie more in emotions more closely connected to human welfare or emotional well-being (for example Diener and Larsen 1993). In this regard, for example, a case could be made for happiness as a fundamental emotion related to the purchase of goods and services, in particular, and emotional well-being, in general (Bagozzi 1999). Finally, recent research shows that emotions are important in building and maintaining connections between brands and consumers and relationships with marketer (for example Fournier 1998).

Social bases of emotions

Although people can experience emotions privately, such as in response to physical danger, a case can be made that emotions are most often interpersonal or group-based responses. Unfortunately, the vast majority of research into emotional behaviour has had an individualistic slant to it (cf. Parkinson 1995). Marketing relationships seem to be contexts where more social conceptualizations of emotions would be worth pursuing. For example, Ruth et al. (1999) review studies where discrete emotions are central in gift-exchanges, and they show how appraisals lead to emotions and how emotions relate to interpersonal relationships and disposition of gifts. Trust and commitment are important variables in the maintenance of marketer–customer relationships (for example Moorman et al. 1992; Garbarino and Johnson 1999). A related area in need of study is the management of emotions by organizations and by the self (for example Hochschild 1983; Bagozzi 1992; Locke 1996). Cultural aspects of emotions deserve further inquiry, too (for example Markus and Shinobu 1994).

One aspect of the social side to emotions can be seen in the functioning of empathy and its relationship to emotions (for example Hoffman 2000). In an investigation of pro-social consequences of negative emotions, Bagozzi and Moore (1994) explored the role of emotions and empathy on decisions to give help to abused children. In Study 1, the effects of a negative emotional-appeal ad were compared with those of a rational-appeal ad; in Study 2, the effects of three levels of intensity of negative-emotion appeals were examined. The negative emotional ads featured a young boy in his home running away from his father in terror. Both studies demonstrated that four negative emotions (anger, sadness, fear, tension) and four aspects of empathy (perspective taking, compassion/pity, protection motivation, fantasy elaboration) mediated the effects of viewing negative emotional ads on decisions to help. Stronger felt negative emotions in the audience led to greater feelings of empathy, and this, in turn, enhanced the decision to help victims of child abuse. It would also be useful to investigate the role of such self-conscious social emotions as pride, guilt, shame, envy, embarrassment, and social anxiety in consumer behaviour (cf. Verbeke and Bagozzi 2000, 2001a, 2001b, 2001c).

Suggested readings

Cohen, J.B. and Areni, C.S. (1991) Affect and consumer behavior, in T.S. Robertson and H.H. Kasarjian (eds) *Handbook of Consumer Behavior*. Englewood Cliffs, NJ: Prentice-Hall. A thorough and conceptually well-thought-out review of the literature prior to 1990.

Lazarus, R.S. (1991) *Emotion and Adaptation*. New York: Oxford University Press. One of the fathers of appraisal theory gives a comprehensive analysis of emotions.

Lewis, M. and Haviland-Jones, J.M. (eds) (2000) *Handbook of Emotions*. New York: Guilford. Provides introductions and overviews of emotion including historical, philosophical and biological perspectives, as well as treatments of many discrete emotion categories.

Oatley, K. (1992) *Best Laid Schemes: The Psychology of Emotions*. Cambridge: Cambridge University Press. A wonderful introduction to emotional research that not only highlights the author's planning and communicative perspective on the field but also weaves in insights from literature, cognitive science and other fields.

Parkinson, B. (1995) *Ideas and Realities of Emotion*. London: Routledge. A thorough review of the literature that is mindful of social constructivist and social aspects of emotion.

4

From cognitive processes, attitudes and emotions to action

The study of consumer behaviour is a fascinating topic, and many have been content with limiting inquiry to what goes on inside the head and body of the consumer, so to speak. Indeed, most research to date has dealt with the bases for actions taken by consumers (for example information processing) but not much on the actions, per se, and how actions are produced. Nevertheless, interest is budding into the examination of what might be termed, 'consumer action', which exists in two forms. *Personal* consumer action refers to a singular human being, with consumption goals of their own, who acts so as to achieve these goals (Bagozzi and Dholakia 1999). *Social* consumer action designates a group or collectivity acting to achieve its consumption goals, wherein members jointly hold the group goal and agree in a particular way to do their parts to achieve the goal (Bagozzi 2000a). In this chapter, we consider both aspects of consumer action. Note, too, that consumer action can be studied from the point of view of dyadic interactions or networks of interactions. One way to do this is by scrutinizing the actions and reactions of people in a relationship, as well as intrapersonal processes for the participants. Dyadic interactions thus may be studied from the point of view of personal consumer action in relation to another person (for example a salesperson).

What is an action?

Consumer action is obviously an important phenomenon to be explained. We might begin by defining consumer action as what a consumer does that can be observed and verified intersubjectively. By observed, we mean that which a person can perceive in or by a consumer, where this occurs either directly through one or more of the five senses or indirectly by use of sense extending instruments. Up to this point, and in the title to this monograph, we have used the term, behaviour, broadly and loosely. So let us now make a clear distinction between behaviour and action. Philosophers sometimes speak of narrow and broad behaviour (Mele 1992):

> Narrow behavior is mere bodily motion, in abstraction from its causes and effects; broad behavior is richer. Representative instances include an agent's unlocking his office door, making up his bed, and eating his Wheaties.
>
> (Mele 1992: 18)

Action is generally identified with the second sense of behaviour: broad behaviour. Many philosophers construe action as bodily movements caused by mental states or events (Bishop 1989). Aristotle nicely captured this perspective long ago: 'the origin of action – its efficient, not its final cause – is choice, and that of choice is desire and reasoning with a view to an end' (*Nicomachean Ethics* 1139ª31–2). There are many complex and contentious issues in the philosophy of action concerning mental causation, intentionality, trying and acts of will. We cannot do justice to these topics in this monograph and merely alert the reader to the importance of being mindful of the conceptual and logical foundations of the variables and processes considered herein. We believe that, as the social psychology of consumer behaviour matures, more attention will be given in the future to metaphysical and epistemological subjects, in general, and the philosophy of mind and the philosophy of action, in particular.

With this as background, we can identify three varieties of consumer action that serve as explananda for consumer researchers. One is the *physiological responses* consumers produce in relation to consumption decisions. These might include skin conductance, hormonal changes, neural activity, heart rate, seemingly imperceptible movements in facial muscles (for example Cacioppo et al. 1986b) and other biological or electro-biochemical changes of the body. Physiological responses might be studied in their own right or as markers of decision making or other internal mental states or processes.

A second class of consumer action for study are *overt movements* of the body produced instantaneously at the end of decision making or seemingly simultaneously with decision making and as a means to achieving a specific goal. For example, a thirsty consumer approaches a soft-drink vending machine, puts money in the slot, and pushes a button selecting a preferred brand. Such immediate actions represent common consumption phenomena to be explained. In some cases, simple observed muscle movements might be actions for study, if, for example, they reflect an emotional response to a brand or product (for example Ekman 1993).

The third class of consumer action concerns *purposive action extended in time* and consists of two subtypes. One involves bodily movements directed at achieving a goal, but, unlike overt movements following immediately upon decision making, occurs after some delay. In such cases, one or more instrumental acts or goal-directed behaviours must be activated and co-ordinated at some future opportune time, and various post-decision deliberative processes (for example planning, monitoring of progress, overcoming impediments, resisting temptations) must be conducted to support goal striving. A second subtype of action entails what philosophers have termed 'trying', and serves as a bridge or transition between internal decision-making processes and overt movements or action of the type described above. Some philosophers appear to include intention, volition, effort, and even simple bodily movements under the umbrella of 'trying' (for example Hornsby 1980; Pietroski 2000). We turn now to contemporary models of action that have been applied frequently to consumer behaviour.

Three leading theories of action

The theory of reasoned action

The **theory of reasoned action** (TRA) is a parsimonious explanation of action and has had wide currency in psychology, as well as other basic and applied disciplines (Fishbein and Ajzen 1975; Ajzen and Fishbein 1980; Sheppard et al. 1988; van den Putte 1993). Under the TRA, action is hypothesized to be a direct function of a person's intentions (see Figure 4.1, panel a). Fishbein and Ajzen maintain that the TRA applies to behaviours under volitional control, by which the authors mean the following:

> [P]eople can easily perform these behaviors, if they are inclined to do so (Ajzen, 1985, p. 12). [W]hen one is asked about performing a behavior that is completely under one's own volitional control, one typically believes that one can, and will, do whatever one intends or tries to do.
> (Fishbein and Stasson 1990: 177)

The authors go on to claim that the TRA applies to a wide range of actions: '[W]e make the assumption that most actions of relevance are under volitional control' (Ajzen and Fishbein 1980: 5).

Ajzen and Fishbein (1980: 41) do not say much, if anything, about what they mean by volitional control and how intention influences actions, except to say that 'intention is the immediate determinant of behavior'. We will have more to say below about how intentions (and related volitional variables) actuate actions, when we critique the leading theories of action and propose alternatives. Likewise, the meaning of the concept, intention, remains undeveloped in the theory of reasoned action, with Ajzen and Fishbein (1980) relying on an operational definition. Namely, for them, intention is the likelihood that one intends to do something (Ajzen and Fishbein 1980: ch. 4). In other words, Ajzen and Fishbein regard intentions

(a) The theory of reasoned action

(b) The theory of planned behaviour

(c) The MODE model

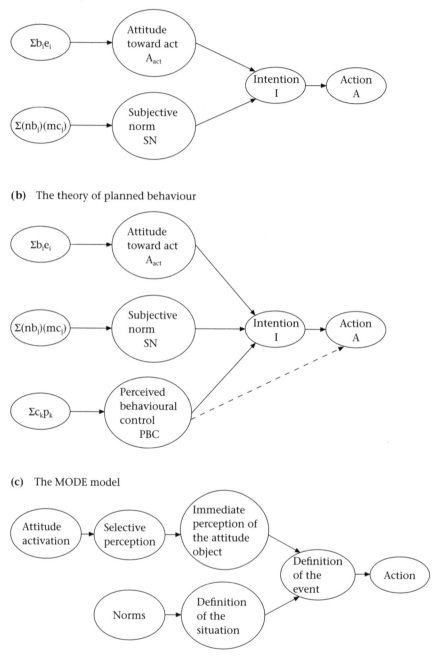

Figure 4.1 Three leading theories of action

as self-predictions or expectations that one will act (cf. Bagozzi et al. 1989). We shall have more to say about deeper and broader senses of intentions below.

Given that intentions cause actions under the TRA, the next issue to address is what influences intentions. Here the theory asserts that one's intention to act is an additive function of one's attitude toward the act and the felt normative pressure ('subjective norm') to act (see Figure 4.1, panel a). Subjective norm is defined as one's 'perception of the social pressure . . . to perform or not perform' the action (Ajzen and Fishbein 1980: 6). These determinants of intentions, in turn, are functions of expectancy-value judgements. That is, beliefs about the consequences of acting and evaluations of these consequences produce attitude, and **normative beliefs** (nb) about the expectations of others and one's **motivation to comply** (mc) with these others determine subjective norm.

The heart of the TRA is intention and its proximal antecedents, which can be depicted through the following regression equation:

$$I = \alpha + \beta_1 A_{act} + \beta_2 SN + e$$

where I = intention to act, A_{act} = attitude toward the act, SN = subjective norm, α is an intercept and e an error term, and β_1 and β_2 are empirically inferred regression weights reflecting the respective effects of A_{act} and SN on I. An underlying assumption in the TRA is that I is sufficient for explaining action, and A_{act} and SN are sufficient for explaining I. In turn, A_{act} and SN are hypothesized to depend on behavioural beliefs (that is, the perceived likelihood of certain outcomes occurring, if one were to act) and normative beliefs (that is, the perceived likelihood certain specific individuals think they should/should not act), respectively. Ajzen and Fishbein (1980: ch. 7) maintain that action is 'ultimately determined' by a person's beliefs and their subsequent effects on A_{act} and SN, which, in turn, influence I and through I, action.

Ajzen and Fishbein (1980) identify a number of 'external variables' that they claim have only indirect effects, if at all, on action, through the variables shown in Figure 4.1, panel a: demographic variables (for example age, gender, occupation, socio-economic status, religion, education), attitudes toward targets (for example people, institutions, objects, brands, services) and personality traits (for example introversion–extraversion, self-esteem, **need for cognition**). The effects of external variables are posited to occur in one or both of two ways. One is a direct effect on beliefs, evaluations, or motivation to comply with the wishes of specific referents. The second is by influencing β_1 and/or β_2 in the equation above, thereby modulating the relative effects of A_{act} and SN on I. Some support exists for the indirect effects of external variables on I or action (for example Loken 1983), but as we will see later, direct effects have been frequently found, bringing into question the sufficiency of the TRA.

The theory of planned behaviour

For actions not completely under volitional control, Ajzen (1985, 1991; Ajzen and Madden 1986) modified the TRA to include perceived behavioural control (PBC) as an additional predictor of both I and action (see Figure 4.1, panel b). PBC is defined as 'the person's belief as to how easy or difficult performance of the behavior is likely to be' (Ajzen and Madden 1986: 457). Ajzen never elaborated on what volitional and non-volitional actions are, so we will temporarily suspend judgement on whether action can be non-volitional or even partially volitional, until we present a critique later. For now, we consider how PBC is claimed to produce its effects. The general idea is that, because behaviours are goals in people's minds, subject to interference or uncertainty, PBC serves to capture the extent to which decision makers take into account problematic personal and situational factors that interfere with or promote action. How PBC does this has not been specified much by Ajzen or others.

The linkage between PBC and I might be interpreted as follows. People will intend to perform a behaviour to the degree that they believe that they have control over the action. But why should mere perceived control influence a decision? Ajzen is silent on this issue. PBC seems totally cognitive and lacking in motivation, yet researchers have ignored this question and presumed that the oft observed empirical association between PBC and I implies causation.

The connection between PBC and action rests, not on a psychological interpretation, but on a physical one (Ajzen and Madden 1986: 459). Ajzen maintains that it is actual control that matters. That is, it is actual control over internal and external factors that could interfere with or facilitate behavioural performance that directly affects behaviour. Thus, PBC is a proxy for the direct physical control one actually has in a given situation. The dashed arrow in Figure 4.1, panel b, is intended to convey the physical effect of actual control on action. A problem arises with Ajzen's interpretation of the effect of actual control on action. Is actual control constituted by, or the result of, volition (for example one's intention)? If the latter, why does not the **theory of planned behaviour** (TPB) have a path from I to PBC such that one intends to do whatever it takes to actuate actual control and this, in turn, results in another action, the focal action displayed in the theory. Or perhaps another intention could be posited to produce actual control. If actual control is a volitional state, what exactly does this mean, and how does it cause the action? The theory is vague on these issues.

Under the TPB, PBC is taken to be a function of the sum of products of (a) beliefs that one has access to factors needed to perform a behaviour, times (b) the perceived power of the factors in contributing to the behaviour (see c_k and p_k, respectively, in Figure 4.1, panel b). The factors taken into account in c_k and p_k include such instances as personal skills, knowledge, opportunities to act and anticipated impediments to action. For example, your decision to exercise tomorrow might depend, in part, on the perceived likelihood that it will rain then, weighted by the extent that you feel that rain would thwart your plans.

Some confusion exists on what PBC actually means. Ajzen (1991) and Eagly and Chaiken (1993: 187) take PBC to be essentially the same as self-efficacy, which Bandura (1994) defines as the confidence one has that he/she can perform a particular action. In contrast, Armitage and Conner (1999) argued and found, in their study of intentions to eat a low-fat diet, that self-efficacy and PBC were distinct and had independent effects on intentions. This suggests that self-efficacy and PBC are different facets of decision making in goal contexts. We shall see below that the seemingly similar concepts as **outcome expectancies** or expectations of success and failure constitute additional reasons for acting or not acting in decision making, related to personal control issues. Still another approach to PBC was taken by Bagozzi et al. (2001c) who conceived of PBC as resistance to temptation, as operationalized by a 14-item scale in a study of dieting.

The TPB has been applied in many contexts. For example, Conner and Sparks (1996) summarize the use of the TPB in such areas as smoking behaviours, alcohol consumption, sexual behaviours, health screening attendance, exercise, food choice, breast/testicle self-examination and other actions. East (1997: 140) lists additional TPB studies covering such topics as blood donation, engaging in collective action, recycling, internet use, accident avoidance behaviour, buying gifts, making investments and consumer complaining. Armitage and Conner (2001) further report the use of the TPB across 154 applications in their meta-analysis.

The MODE model

The TRA and TPB are largely rational accounts of decision making in that they appear to rest on the notion that consumers deliberate (for example process information, form beliefs, weigh pros and cons) before deciding to act. Fazio (1986, 1990) argued that such deliberative models apply only to the extent that people have the opportunity and motivation to process information, arrive at an attitude and make other judgements, and decide to act on the basis of one's attitudes and judgements. He proposed an alternative model based on the notion that behaviour is sometimes spontaneously produced when an attitude is activated. An attitude can be automatically activated from memory by observation of either an attitude object or cues associated with the object, depending on the extent of attitude accessibility (that is, the strength of association between an attitude object and an evaluation in memory). Fazio termed his model the **MODE model** (motivation and opportunity as determinants of how attitudes influence behaviour).

Figure 4.1, panel c, shows the MODE model. Once an attitude is activated, this leads to selective perception of features of the attitude object that are congruent with one's attitude. Perceptions of the attitude object influence one's definition of the event or occasion for acting. Norms also influence this definition of the event through an interpretation of the larger social situation in which the event is embedded. Action then immediately follows. As Fazio (1986: 237) conceives the process: 'once activated, the attitude biases perceptions of the object in the immediate situation, and behavior simply follows from these perceptions without any necessary conscious reasoning'. Notice that action is spontaneous in the MODE model, with no deliberations occurring either for attitude or subjective norm formation or for decision making or intention formation.

Fazio's conceptualization of the automatic activation of attitudes shows some similarity to Fiske and Pavelchak's (1986) notion of category-based evaluations wherein an attitude object is stored in memory as a category and linked to both its attributes and other object categories, as well as affective tags, which represent stored evaluations of object categories. When a person is exposed to an instance of a stored category (for example they see an ad for a product), they may access the stored affective tag to arrive at an evaluation, depending on the degree of fit between the instance and the category. This direct activation of an evaluation is termed category-based processing by Fiske and Pavelchak (1986). For example, I may have a well-formed attitude toward watching 'horror movies', such that the idea or category of horror movies is stored in memory and connected to a positive feeling therein. Then as I glance through the entertainment section of the newspaper and come across an advertisement of a new rendition of *Dracula*, my positive attitude toward horror movies will be activated, a rosy picture of the new film induced, and I begin to take steps to go to the cinema forthwith.

Parallel to Fazio's contrast of automatic attitude activation to deliberative processing, Fiske and Pavelchak (1986) oppose category-based processing with piecemeal-based processing, by which they mean a person forms an evaluation of an object by appraising and integrating evaluations associated with the attributes or characteristics of the object. As noted later in this book, Sujan (1985) used these ideas to explain differences in processing of products by novices and experts. Note also the similarity between central versus peripheral processing (for example Petty and Cacioppo 1986) and systematic versus heuristic processing (for example Chaiken 1980) of persuasive communication, on the one hand, as discussed in the next chapter, and Fazio's (1986, 1990) and Fiske and Pavelchak's (1986) approaches to attitude. Only Fazio, however, considers explicitly the effect of attitude on behaviour, per se.

In sum, we see a distinction between conscious, deliberative processing models, on the one hand, and non-conscious, automatic processing models, on the other hand. This contrast may be a bit strained, however, when one realizes that under some condition A_{act}, SN and PBC might be regarded as stored summaries of their presumed, respective information processing or conditioned bases, to be retrieved or activated on a later occasion. Also Bargh et al. (1992) have shown that even weak attitudes can be activated automatically, not merely strong ones, bringing into question the argument that attitude accessibility is the basis for automatic activation of attitudes. It may be, too, that people, without a well-formed or stored attitude, nevertheless, are capable of having an attitude based on the information at hand or on an intuitive sense of their attitude at the moment. We might view our own and others' attitudes as tentative hypotheses, evolving evaluations, or temporary judgements one has that are adjusted, updated or discarded as the need arises. Other attitudes are long-standing evaluations that are actuated or retrieved on demand or in the right circumstances. Still other attitudes may be constructed thoughtfully anew with considerable processing and reflection. The above speculations suggest that researchers need to continue investigating the conditions governing attitude acquisition and change, as well as individual differences in the formation and use of attitudes (see also emerging research on implicit attitudes, for example, Maison et al. 2001).

Shortcomings with contemporary theories and three alternatives

The theory of trying

Bagozzi and Warshaw (1990) suggested that many consumer actions can be studied from the perspective of *trying* to act. The idea is that decision makers often realize that performance of an intended act is problematic in their own minds, because they recognize either that they have personal shortcomings (for example limited resources, weakness of will) or situational conditions might thwart action (for example a proposed shopping trip may be uncertain because of anticipated bad weather). In sum, many actions are goals in people's minds. How many actions are so construed? Ajzen (1985) claims that virtually all behaviours are goals because performance of even the most mundane act is subject to forestalment by some unforeseen event. We are not so sure about this conclusion and feel that at least some actions are viewed by consumers as largely unproblematic or are taken for granted. In any case, the relative incidence of goal-directed consumer behaviours, which particular acts are perceived as goals, and how individual consumers differ in this regard are important topics for future study.

To fulfil one's consumption goals a consumer must see their own action as a purposive endeavour where foresight and effort are needed. For example, consumers often are at a loss for what to purchase as a gift for a special person's birthday. To find an appropriate gift, they may see their task as one of trying to do the things needed to accomplish this goal. This might mean deciding to embark on a trip to visit a shopping area, identifying a set of stores to browse, deciding on a rough estimate on how much to spend, reflecting upon things the recipient of the gift likes to do or experience, and so on. Figure 4.2, panel a, presents the theory of trying (TT), which attempts to account for such a 'trying to consume', and in this case might involve the

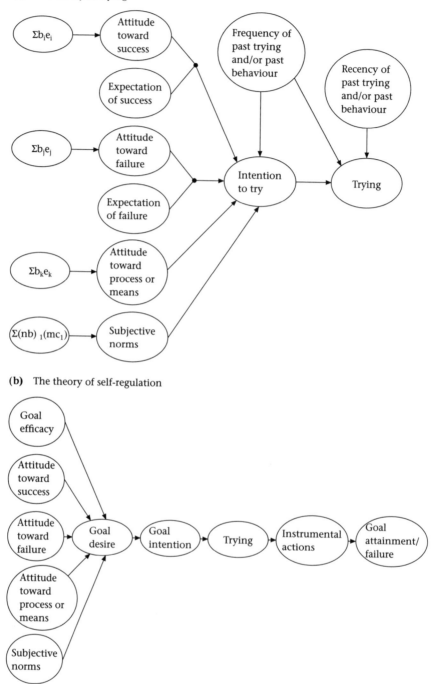

Figure 4.2 Recent models overcoming limitations in contemporary theories of consumer action

instrumental goal of acting so as to purchase a gift, with the further goal in mind to express one's caring and friendship and celebrate this with another person and friends (Bagozzi and Warshaw 1990; Bagozzi and Edwards 1998). Consistent with the TRA and TPB, the TT posits that intentions, particularly intentions to try, are direct antecedents of trying. Unlike the TRA and TPB, the TT construes attitudes as multidimensional reactions to the consequences of acting, in terms of the goals for which trying serves (see discussion on multidimensional goal-directed attitudes in Chapter 2). Thus, it is hypothesized that three attitudinal reactions are formed (in the case of a new attitude) or activated (in the case of an existing attitude): attitudes toward pursuing a goal and succeeding (A_s), attitudes toward pursuing a goal but failing (A_f) and attitudes toward the means or process of goal pursuit (A_p). Each of these components of attitudes might be a function of separate expectancy-value responses (see Figure 4.2, panel a) or functions of either classes of appraisals or hierarchical arrangements or reasons in means-end chains (not shown in Figure 4.2; see Chapter 2). The original TT included an attitude toward trying as a mediator between A_s, A_f and A_p, on the one hand, and intentions, on the other hand, but this is omitted from Figure 4.2, for simplicity.

Bagozzi and Warshaw (1990) also proposed that consumer expectations (E_s and E_f) moderate the effects of A_s and A_f on intentions (see Figure 4.2, panel a). In particular, consumer expectations of success interact with A_s, and expectations of failure interact with A_f, to influence intentions. Expectations of success and failure are similar to Bandura's (1994) ideas on outcome expectancy. Note, however, that E_s and E_f are different than PBC under the TPB and Bandura's (1994) better known concept of self-efficacy. The sense of personal control over internal and external impediments and the self-confidence that one has the ability to act are major determinants of decisions, but it is important to realize that, in one sense, E_s and E_f are more fundamental or determinative in that they can be conceived as results of PBC and self-efficacy and thus function as more proximal influences of decisions (in interaction with A_s and A_f, respectively). Carver and Scheier (1998: 204–8) recently exposued a somewhat similar conclusion and noted further that perceived personal control can be detrimental to action in certain instances (for example if it increases distress).

A third addition to attitude theory that Bagozzi and Warshaw (1990) suggested concerns the incorporation of prior learning and past behaviour in the explanation of intentions and trying. A number of studies in the early years of tests of both the TRA (for example Bentler and Speckart 1979, 1981; Bagozzi 1981b; Fredericks and Dossett 1983; Wittenbraker et al. 1983; Bagozzi and Warshaw 1992; Bagozzi and Kimmel 1995), and the TPB (for example Beck and Ajzen 1991; Ajzen and Driver 1992; Bagozzi and Kimmel 1995; Norman and Smith 1995; Norman and Conner 1996; Leone et al. 1999) found that past behaviour was a significant predictor of intentions and/or subsequent behaviour. This brings into question the sufficiency of the TRA and TPB, because past behaviour fails to work through the variables in the theories, as Fishbein and Ajzen hypothesized, but instead has direct effects on intentions and behaviour.

Bagozzi and Warshaw (1990) proposed that past behaviour can be partitioned into frequency and recency effects (see Figure 4.2, panel a). The need for separate frequency and recency effects can be seen in everyday behaviour. A person may have a long history of performing a given behaviour without having performed it recently (for example a person who long ago gave up regularly purchasing lottery tickets, after experiencing a string of frustrated hopes) or a person may have recently taken up an activity with no prior experience with it (for example a first-time skier).

The effects of the frequency of performance of past behaviour might be explained as follows (Bagozzi and Warshaw 1990). One way that this happens is when attitudes are not strong functions of past behaviour but past behaviour is a proxy for a stored **script** predisposing one to intend to act or act directly. Also to the extent that attitudes and/or intentions are unclear, ill-formed or unstable, independent effects of the frequency of past behaviour on subsequent behaviour might be expected (for example Bagozzi and Yi 1989). A meta-analysis examined 64 studies and found robust evidence for the impact of frequency of past behaviour on both intentions and future behaviours (Ouellette and Wood 1998). The authors proposed two processes through which frequency of past behaviour guides future behaviour. When a behaviour is well practised in a constant environment, frequency of past behaviour reflects habit strength and therefore has a direct effect on future behaviour. However, when behaviours are not well learned or when they are performed in unstable contexts, frequency of past behaviour contributes directly to intentions because 'people are likely to form favourable intentions about acts they have frequently performed in the past' (Ouellette and Wood 1998: 56). A somewhat similar perspective has been put forth by Aarts and Dijksterhuis (2000) who maintain that habit is a form of goal-directed automatic action, which is activated spontaneously when relevant cues are present (see also Verplanken et al. 1998; Sheeran and Orbell 1999a).

The recency of past behaviour performance should influence future behaviour to the extent that availability and anchoring/adjustment biases occur in information processing (for example Tversky and Kahneman 1974) and to the degree that an activity, whether established or not, has been recently initiated. Remembrance of the recent initiation of an activity may carry implicit information about intentions, over and above the degree to which intentions or attitudes are accessible to conscious awareness (Greenwald and Banaji 1995; Bargh and Barndollar 1996; Verplanken et al. 1997). Recency of past behaviour may serve as an indirect indicator that an intention has been activated and therefore be positively associated with subsequent performance of the behaviour.

A question that needs further thought is how should we interpret studies including past behaviour as antecedents of intentions and action. Ajzen

(1991) criticized the use of past behaviour on the grounds that it offers no explanatory content, although he allowed that past behaviour provides methodological control in tests of the TRA and TPB: 'past behaviour can be used to test the sufficiency of any model designed to predict future behavior' (Ajzen 1991: 202). Sutton (1998) emphasized the need to distinguish between prediction and explanation and offered many reasons why the TRA and TPB do not always predict as well as one might like them to do. These reasons include the possibility that intentions change before the occasion for action occurs, intentions are often provisional, measures in the TRA and TPB do not correspond with respect to action, context, target or time, measurement scales do not correspond in format, the number of response categories conflicts between measures of intention and behaviour, random error is present in measures, restrictions in range of measures occur, marginal distributions in measures do not match, and other causes of behaviour exist but are not considered. An important point of consideration is that too many studies have measured behaviour contemporaneously with intentions, attitudes, subjective norms and perceived behavioural control, and past behaviour has too often been restricted to retrospective self-reports also measured contemporaneously with the aforementioned variables (Sutton 1994). This makes conclusions with respect to prediction and causality tenuous.

In sum, the TT reconceptualizes the form of attitudes to reflect three aspects of goal attainment/goal pursuit (success, failure, pursuit) and introduces new variables (expectations of success and failure, recency and frequency of past behaviour, and trying) in an attempt to better explain decision making and action. To date, a number of studies have used the TT to investigate such topics as regulating hypertension (Taylor et al. 2001), studying for exams (Leone and Perugini 2000), adopting new computer technologies (Bagozzi et al. 1992c), low-risk single-occasion drinking (Murgraff et al. 2000), exercising and dieting (Bagozzi and Kimmel 1995), losing weight (Bagozzi and Warshaw 1990; Bagozzi and Edwards 1998), achieving goals in experimental tasks (Hinsz and Ployhart 1998), adopting pharmacy services (Odedina et al. 1999) and diet or dieting decisions (Bagozzi et al. 2001c; Capozza and Bagozzi 2001).

The theory of self-regulation

Three additional improvements to the TRA, TPB and TT were suggested by Bagozzi in the theory of self-regulation (TSR) (Bagozzi 1992; Bagozzi and Edwards 1998). Figure 4.2, panel b, shows these, which encompass an expansion of the meaning of trying, the introduction of desires as mediators between the antecedents in the TT and intentions, and the addition of **goal efficacy**.

Bagozzi and Warshaw (1990) originally conceived of trying as a singular subjective state summarizing the extent to which a person believes they have tried or will 'try' to act. Bagozzi (1992) expanded the notion of trying to embrace a set of psychological and physical processes intervening between intentions and goal achievement/failure: planning, monitoring of progress toward a goal, guidance and control activities, commitment to the goal and one's intention, and effort. A portion of these trying processes was tested in a study of body weight loss/maintenance (Bagozzi and Edwards 1998). Here trying was operationalized as separate mental and physical activities used to initiate and regulate instrumental actions (that is, exercising and dieting) to achieve one's weight loss/maintenance goals (see also Bagozzi et al. 1990, 1998). The trying activities included maintaining willpower and self-discipline, devoting time for planning with respect to the instrumental acts, and expending physical energy in goal pursuit. In a study of self-regulation of hypertension, Taylor et al. (2001) operationalized trying in the senses of (a) devoting time to planning with respect to reducing/maintaining blood pressure, (b) expending mental/physical energy to reduce/maintain blood pressure, (c) maintaining will power to reduce/maintain blood pressure, and (d) sustaining self-discipline to reduce/maintain blood pressure. In still another investigation of aspects of trying, Bagozzi and Edwards (2000) showed how appraisals of means (self-efficacy, outcome expectancies and affect towards the means) and strength of impediments interact to regulate goal-directed behaviours in the pursuit of weight loss/maintenance goals. The above studies showed that trying is an important mediator and initiator of goal-directed behaviours (see also discussion of the **model of goal-directed behaviour** on pp. 95–6).

An important issue for further study is how exactly to conceive of trying. Bagozzi and Edwards (1998) defined trying as mental and physical activities leading up to and regulating the instrumental acts producing goal attainment/failure. But the envelope could be extended to cover the instrumental acts themselves, as well as intention and volition. The line between intentions, volition, trying and goal-directed behaviours is difficult to draw, and it may be that 'trying' is an omnibus term implicating intentions, planning, monitoring of goal progress, guidance and control activities, maintenance of commitment, willpower and initiation of instrumental acts. If so, emphasis needs to be placed on the specific mental states and events and on the physical activities comprising trying, as well as their structure and interaction, in any particular context. It is these details, not the omnibus term, that are crucial for understanding how decisions are transformed into action and goal attainment. Yet, in some research contexts, people do seem to have an overall subjective sense of 'trying', that may warrant separate study.

A second contribution under the TSR is the importation of desire as a key mediator between the antecedents listed in the left-hand portion of Figure 4.2, panel b, and intentions. It can be argued that the TRA, TPB and TT fail to consider how intentions become energized (Calder and Ross 1973: 7; Bagozzi 1992; Fazio 1995: 271–2). Attitudes, SNs and PBC provide reasons for acting, it is claimed, but do not incorporate explicit motivational content needed to induce an intention to act. Similar to Gollwitzer's designation for wants and wishes in his action phases model (for example Gollwitzer et al.

1990: 1119), Bagozzi (1992: 184–6) proposed that desires provide the motivational impetus for intentions and suggested that A_{act}, SN and PBC work through desires enroute to influencing intentions. This happens in one of two ways. With volitive desires (Davis 1984a), A_{act}, SN and PBC provide reasons for acting that a decision maker takes into account to form a self-commitment to act. Some philosophers maintain that desires have a particular kind of relationship to intentions in the sense that, once one is aware of and accepts one's desire to act, this will motivate the person to form an intention. Davis (1984b: 53) calls this the 'connection condition' for intentions (see also Frankfurt 1988). This functioning of desire is similar to Searle's (1983) notion of a mental state (for example intention) coming to cause action by representing itself in causing the action. With appetitive desires (Davis 1984a), A_{act}, SN and PBC serve as catalysts to release or free-up a hidden or latent desire related to such biological needs as food or sex, in contrast to their arousing function for volitive desires (Bagozzi 1992). Further arguments for the conceptual distinction between desires and intentions, as well as empirical support for convergent and discriminant validity of their measures, can be found in Bratman (1987), Bagozzi (1992), Mele (1992), Bagozzi and Kimmel (1995), Malle and Knobe (1997), Leone et al. (1999), Perugini and Conner (2000) and Perugini and Bagozzi (2001a, 2001b, 2001c). Empirical support for the mediating role of desires can be found in Bagozzi and Kimmel (1995), Bagozzi and Edwards (1998), Leone et al. (1999), Perugini and Conner (2000), Dholakia et al. (2001), Perugini and Bagozzi (2001a), Taylor et al. (2001) and Bagozzi and Dholakia (2002).

Perugini and Conner (2000) further distinguished between goal desires and behavioural desires, where the latter can be considered an extrinsic desire, that is, 'a desire for something for its believed conduciveness to something else that one desires' (Mele 1995: 391). In their study of body weight regulation and studying effort, Perugini and Conner (2000) found that measures of goal desires and behavioural desires achieved convergent and discriminant validity. In addition, goal desires were the most important predictor of behavioural desires, compared to the other antecedents in the model.

The final new variable introduced by the TSR is goal efficacy. Bagozzi and Edwards (1998) defined goal efficacy as the perceived likelihood of goal achievement, given that one decides to try to achieve a goal. It is thus similar to goal outcome expectancies or expectations of success. Similar to Carver and Scheier (1998: 204), Bagozzi and Edwards argued that goal efficacy is a more fundamental and proximal antecedent of decision making, in the sense that self-efficacy and perceived behavioural control might work through goal efficacy to influence decisions.

Consumption as a goal-directed activity

An important shortcoming of both the TRA and TPB is that neither theory explicitly models aspects of goal setting and goal striving. In Chapter 2 on attitudes, we considered a number of ways that goal setting is done. Recall that it is useful to conceive of a three-tiered hierarchy of goals that underlie consumer behaviour (see Figure 2.4 in Chapter 2). At the centre of the hierarchy is one's focal goal, which answers the question, 'What is it for which I strive?' The focal goal is dependent on subordinate goals, which answer the question, 'How can I achieve that for which I strive?' The raison d'être for one's focal goal lies in its contributions to the achievement of superordinate goals, which answer the question, 'Why do I want to achieve that for which I strive?' For example, my focal goal 'to prevent gum disease' may be accomplished by purchasing and using dental floss, and tartar and plaque control mouth rinses, as well as by visiting the dentist quarterly (these latter means are my subordinate goals). Preventing gum disease may, in turn, satisfy higher aims related to enhancing my appearance, avoiding future pain and inconvenience, saving money, and in general contributing to health and longevity and a sense of well-being (my superordinate goals). Figure 2.3 in Chapter 2 illustrates a superordinate goal structure for losing/ maintaining one's body weight. Two methods for ascertaining goals and their interrelationships were discussed in Chapter 2: namely, categorization theory (for example Barsolou 1991) and means-end chain theory (for example Reynolds and Gutman 1988; Pieters et al. 1995; Bagozzi and Edwards 1998; Bagozzi and Dabholkar 2000). Barsolou's (1991) categorization theory and means-end chain theory address the topic of goal setting, which is not considered in the TRA, TPB, TT and TSR.

Moreover, the TRA and TPB do not investigate goal striving but rather presume that intentions lead directly to action. The TRA and TPB fail to specify how intentions influence action and what psychological processes follow intention formation, if any. Goal-striving processes are thus ignored.

Figure 4.3 presents an outline of how goal-setting and goal-striving processes might be conceived in consumer behaviour (Bagozzi and Dholakia 1999: 20). Consumption as a goal-directed activity begins with goal setting, which involves decision-making processes and can figuratively be thought to answer two broad questions: 'What are the goals I can pursue, and why do I want or not want to pursue them?' Most information processing theories of consumer behaviour have taken the motivation or goal of consumers as a given.

Given a sufficiently strong desire to pursue a goal, actual goal pursuit will commence in one of three conditions. Sometimes for frequently performed consumption activities, goal pursuit is activated more or less automatically by responses to learned cues, and little conscious processing is involved (for example running a credit card through the scanner at the supermarket checkout counter). This might be labelled 'habitual goal-directed consumer behaviour'. Habitual behaviour must begin somewhere, of course. In general, its origins reside in prior deliberative processing or learning shaped by either classical or operant conditioning or in some combination of deliberative processing and conditioning. When acquired, however, habitual behaviour

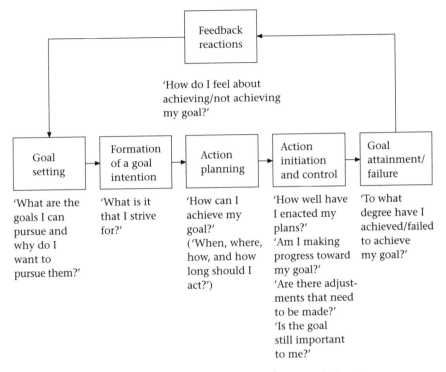

Figure 4.3 Goal setting and goal pursuit in consumer behaviour

is initiated and performed with little conscious self-regulation of the sort on which we focus in this monograph. Another way that goal pursuit occurs, at least in a minimal way, is with impulsive acts. By definition, impulsive acts do not entail prior deliberation or planning, but they do involve some awakening of a need or desire that quickly becomes a goal to be achieved through minimal goal-directed activities.

The final class of actual goal-pursuit activities, and the ones we emphasize herein, are those that are clearly volitional in nature. As we show in Figure 4.3, goal pursuit is initiated volitionally with the formation of a **goal intention**, which answers the question, 'What is it for which I strive?' Goal intentions are targeted at either specific acts as end performances (for example 'I intend to buy a Sony DVD player tonight') or particular outcomes to be achieved through the execution of instrumental acts (for example 'I intend to lose two pounds by exercising vigorously with my ProForm treadmill during the next week'). Goal intentions directed at end performances have been studied extensively in consumer behaviour with the TRA, in which they are termed 'behavioural intentions' because the targets of the intentions are actions. Goal intentions directed at outcomes sometimes have been studied with the TRA, but as the authors of the theory have emphasized, the theory is not applicable to outcome or end-state goals (Ajzen and Fishbein 1980: 29–30, 111). The present framework is designed in part to apply to such decision-making contexts, as well as contexts in which actions are goals.

Another type of volition that has not been studied systematically by consumer behaviour researchers is the so-called **implementation intention**, which is a person's intention to perform a goal-directed behaviour (for example execute an instrumental act), given that future contingencies occur: 'I intend to do X when situation Y is encountered' (Gollwitzer 1996: 292). For example, an implementation intention to perform a future act in the service of goal achievement might read: 'I intend to withdraw $60 from an automated teller machine (ATM) every time my cash on hand is $10 or less.' An example of an implementation intention to achieve a future goal might read: 'I intend to balance my portfolio of investments next year by adding new growth stocks in high-tech Asian industries as they become available' (see also Verplanken and Faes 1999).

The third stage shown in Figure 4.3, action planning, is also volitional and elaborates further on implementation intentions. Here, focus is on the general question, 'How can I achieve my goal?' and the specific amplifications addressing 'When, where, how and how long should I act in this regard?' (Gollwitzer 1996). The choice of means is an important part of planning (Bagozzi 1992). It is at this stage that specific implementation intentions are formed.

Following planning, actual implementation steps are taken in a fourth stage, labelled 'action initiation and control' in Figure 4.3. Here, delayed intentions are enacted, and goal-directed behaviours are guided. Four questions are addressed: 'Am I making progress toward my goal?', 'How well have I enacted my plans?', 'Are there adjustments that need to be made?' and 'Is the goal still important to me?' Implementation intentions are realized in this stage.

The fifth stage, goal attainment/failure, involves a final comparison of the outcome achieved with a standard or reference value and determination of whether to maintain or increase efforts at goal pursuit or disengage from further efforts (for example Carver and Scheier 1998). Figuratively, the consumer asks: 'To what degree have I achieved/failed to achieve my ends, and should I continue on with or terminate goal striving?'

Finally, for feedback reactions, the discrepancy between a person's goal and its achievement is appraised, and emotional responses are generated, including reactions of satisfaction or dissatisfaction, among others. The question considered here is: 'How do I feel about achieving/not achieving my goal?' Emotional and rational reactions to goal attainment/failure ultimately update the person's knowledge structure about goals, motivation to pursue goals, and other learning with regard to planning, means and implementation. The emotions that follow goal attainment/failure were discussed in

Chapter 3. Much research has gone on in the study of one emotion in this regard, satisfaction, and can be found in Oliver (1997), Johnson (1998) and Johnson and Gustafsson (2000).

Bagozzi and Dholakia (1999) summarize research into goal striving. The early stages of goal striving are set up through intention formation. Both goal and implementation intentions are stored abstractly in declarative memory and must be retrieved before further progress in goal pursuit can occur (Goschke and Kuhl 1996). To realize a goal intention, there must be enactment of a choice of means to pursue the goal and other planning activities. To realise an implementation intention, recognition of execution conditions must occur. The memory processes for both types of intentions involve internalized verbal instructions (for example Diaz and Berk 1992).

Because many consumption decisions are fulfilled at a time quite remote from the point when an intention first was formed, two basic memory processes come into play with delayed intentions. One refers to remembering to perform an action at a future point in time and has come to be known as **prospective memory** (for example Kvavilashvili and Ellis 1996). The other requires remembering the content of the action to perform and the conditions for its execution. This is called 'retrospective memory' in the literature.

Before we consider prospective and retrospective memory in the functioning of intentions, let us consider an example to describe the nature of the processes. On awakening this morning, I find that I am out of breakfast cereal and decide to replenish my 'supplies, as well as purchase ingredients for making my lunches for the rest of the week. I intend to do this later in the afternoon. For this decision to be transformed into action, I must remember at the appropriate time (as I drive home after work and pass the supermarket) that I had formed an intention earlier in the day. This is the recall of my goal intention and is an example of prospective memory. Next, I must recall the content of my decision; that is, I must remember where in the store to go (dairy section, produce area, canned goods shelves and so forth), what to buy (breakfast cereal, sourdough bread, canned tuna, low-fat mayonnaise, fresh fruit) and so on. This is my retrospective memory and, among other things, involves the execution of implementation intentions.

My prospective memory requires that my intention persists, that I am vigilant for external cues, such as the supermarket marquee, or that the intention becomes activated by unplanned stimuli or spontaneously. My retrospective memory requires deliberative and directive cognitive processing or automatic retrieval of plans or executive functions when the prospective memory becomes activated.

Psychologists have begun to uncover important aspects of prospective memory. Goschke and Kuhl (1996), for example, find in their experiments that the contents of prospective memory have stronger and more sustained levels of activation than other non-intention memory content. They also show that intentions facilitate subsequent processing of intention-related information, even when the episodic representation of the intention is not consciously recollected. Finally, Goschke and Kuhl (1996) find that state- versus action-oriented subjects showed stronger persistence of intentions. Ruminations by the former (for example intrusions into memory of previous goal failures) contributed to the persistence, whereas the latter, who tend to act quickly and not become distracted or dwell on failures, deactivated intention-related material to a greater extent.

Kvavilashvili and Ellis (1996) consider further aspects of prospective memory. They discuss different types of prospective memory failures and errors, as well as describe how retrieval contexts prompt delayed intentions.

In mediating between goal intentions and acting upon the goal in question, implementation intentions are thought to perform two functions (Gollwitzer and Brandstätter 1997). Cognitively, implementation intentions provide mental representations of the opportunities implied by the intentions. It is believed that these would 'attract attention, be easily remembered, and be effectively recognised' in a relevant situation (Gollwitzer and Brandstätter 1997: 196). Volitionally, implementation intentions 'create strong mental links between intended situations and behaviours' and 'in the presence of the critical situation, the intended behaviour will be elicited automatically' (Gollwitzer and Brandstätter 1997: 196).

In a series of studies, Gollwitzer and Brandstätter (1997) found that sub- jects' formation of implementation intentions significantly increased the likelihood that goal-directed behaviours were subsequently performed, in comparison to subjects who had only formed goal intentions. This occurred for 'difficult', as opposed to 'easy', personal goals. One explanation the authors gave for their findings was that easy-to-implement goals were likely to have been habitualized, and thus the additional formation of implementation intentions would not have discernible effects on behaviour. But for difficult- to-implement goals, implementation intentions produce the cognitive and volitional qualities noted above, which facilitate action initiation and goal attainment. Orbell et al. (1997) provide a conceptual replication of Gollwitzer and Brandstätter's (1997) study in that they, too, found that implementation intentions increased the likelihood of behavioural enactment. Women who formed an implementation intention were much more likely to perform breast self-examinations than women who formed only goal intentions (64 per cent versus 14 per cent).

Bagozzi and Edwards (2000) showed further how appraisals of means (that is, self-efficacy, outcome expectancies, and affect toward means under con- ditions of weak versus strong impediments) transform goal intentions into goal-directed behaviours. For relatively easy-to-implement goal-directed beha- viours, either self-efficacy, outcome expectancy or affect towards means was sufficient to initiate action. For difficult-to-implement goal-directed behavi- ours, self-efficacy, outcome expectancy, and affect towards means combined multiplicatively (that is, interacted) to initiate action. This study shows that the choice of means is an important activity in planning and initiation of goal-directed behaviours (see also Bagozzi et al. 1992a).

In many cases, especially when there is a time gap between intention formation and action initiation, impediments to the enactment of the actions necessary for goal attainment may occur after the implementation plan has been formed. For example, a store may be stocked out of a favourite brand, a more appealing movie may be discovered playing in the multiplex theatre after the arrival and plan has been made to attend a different movie, or other goal alternatives may be perceived on the surface as more attractive in everyday shopping activities because of new information. In such cases, if the goal is to be achieved, the originally formed goal intention must be maintained and protected from these competing goal alternatives, and implementation plans must be facilitated in a broader process termed 'guidance and control'. Of course, a decision may be made to abandon the goal in favour of another. Processes of self-regulation (or what Kuhl (1984) terms the 'mechanisms of action control') play an important role in this intention maintenance process (see also Kuhl and Beckmann 1994). Carver and Scheier (1998) consider the evaluations people make with regard to progress in goal pursuit. Reactions of doubt and confidence may become important when progress is less than or equal (or greater) than expectations, respectively.

Kuhl (1984) identifies seven volitional self-regulatory processes (that is, those driven by willpower) that, through strategies such as inhibiting the processing of information that supports competing intentions, controlling emotional reactions and maintaining high levels of motivation, protects the chosen intention and implementation plan from being abandoned during the period between intention formation and action initiation. In addition, failure to achieve sub-goals and actual or anticipated extraneous events that threaten plans or goal commitment may result in volitional mechanisms of plan modification. These volitional strategies of self-regulation support and maintain the level of activation of the goal and the plan elements in memory, facilitating subsequent retrieval at the appropriate time. In a study of coupon usage, the relative impact of attitudes on decision making became more important as people became action-oriented, whereas the relative impact of subjective norms on decision making became more important as people became state-oriented (Bagozzi et al. 1992b). Other individual difference variables recently found to affect persistence in goal pursuit include volitional competence (for example Kuhl and Beckmann 1994) and goal orientations (for example Dweck 1991).

Bagozzi and Dholakia (1999) also consider research on action planning. Implementation plans for consumer tasks are likely to vary along several dimensions, depending on the nature and difficulty of the task, as well as the effort anticipated for intention realization. We point out some of the important dimensions, but because little is known about consumer plans, further research must address this issue of plan typologies in greater detail. See Dholakia and Bagozzi (2002) for a recent experiment investigating these processes in a consumer context.

In examining the influence of planning on social behaviour, social psychologists make the distinction between the *content* of plans on the one hand and their *structure* on the other (for example Mischel and Patterson 1976). This provides a convenient distinction to begin to develop a plan typology for consumer tasks. Whereas content refers to the matter contained in the plan, structure pertains to the level of hierarchical organization of the plan. Mischel and Patterson (1976) found that the efficacy of plans depends on both their content and their structure. In their empirical study, temptation-inhibiting plans, which were elaborated in detail, were more successful than task-facilitating elaborated plans in the accomplishment of the goal of self-control.

Furthermore, plan structure can be viewed as having several sub-dimensions. One important sub-dimension of consumer plans is *completeness*, which refers to how fully each individual link in the course of action is specified. We expect that for consumer tasks that are high in salience or difficult to achieve, more complete plans are likely to be formed. A plan to buy a dress for an important party should be formed more completely than one to buy ordinary work clothes.

Closely related to completeness is the sub-dimension of *plan specificity*, which pertains to the various anticipated situational contexts and the specificity of actions to be executed in each context. Specific plans are more likely to be formed in cases in which there is greater certainty about the means to achieve goals, such as purchasing from a store. In cases in which the goal is more difficult and the means uncertain, as in the case of losing weight or quitting smoking, less specific plans are likely to be formed. Highly specific plans are more likely to facilitate intention realization by providing a mechanism to facilitate the retrieval of intentions from memory (Orbell et al. 1997).

Yet another important dimension along which consumer plans vary is *novelty*, which depends on whether the cues and sequences specified are well practised, familiar and reliable for the individual. Novel plans are likely to be especially useful for intention realization.

Implementation plans set the stage for intermediary acts needed to implement a contingent or non-contingent intention. When the instrumental acts have been set in motion, they must be scrutinized to ascertain whether they begin and end when they are supposed to, whether they achieve their objectives, and whether new contingencies, impediments or facilitating factors must be incorporated into the goal-setting process.

The final topic we wish to briefly discuss is whether consumer action is entirely volitional or whether it is possible, as Ajzen (1985, 1991) claims, that the TPB applies to behaviours not totally under volitional control. It is difficult to conceive of any action that is not volitional, for the very meaning of volition implies action caused by mental states or events. Consider two definitions of volition.

Volition is

(a) A mental act of willing or trying, whose presence is sometimes supposed to make the difference between intentional or voluntary action and mere behaviour.

(Blackburn 1994: 395)

(b) The faculty of will; or an item (sometimes alternatively called an act of will) conceived as the product of such a faculty.

In many dualist and empirical accounts of action, volitions are mental items that cause bodily motions on occasions of human agency.

(Honderich 1995: 902)

We would maintain that the vast majority of actions of interest to consumer researchers are volitional and that it does not make sense to claim that some actions are partially under volitional control. Tryings or goal-directed bodily movements are volitional in the senses defined above. This is not to deny that people sometimes try to act but fail to do so, for various reasons. In this case, no action occurs.

Perhaps what Ajzen and others embracing the idea of non-volitional or partially volitional behaviour have in mind is not *action* but *outcomes* or *goal attainment* produced by action. Outcomes or goal attainment are problematic, given trying or goal-directed bodily movements made to produce the outcome or achieve the goal. For example, when I tee-up a golf ball with the aim of hitting it and landing on a par 3 green, achievement of that aim is problematic. But my action – the movement of my body and the golf club in a coordinated way – is not problematic. Of course, these movements can be more or less well done. Theories of action explain fully my initiation and execution of the golf swing but do not fully explain achievement or non-achievement of my goal to hit the ball on the green. The latter depends on such factors beyond my volitional control as the stability of my foot-placement, the absence of unexpected noise and visual distractions, the conditions of the wind, the outcome of my judgement in club selection, the hardness of the green, and so forth. What the theories of action explain are my goal-directed behaviours (for example directed bodily movements) not the downstream outcomes of these behaviours. The former is fully volitional (though it can be misguided, poorly thought out and executed, and so on), the latter is neither volitional nor non-volitional. To predict or understand the latter, we need to investigate consumer action as well as physical and social forces combining with action to produce or fail to produce the sought for result.

Towards an integrative theory of consumer action

With the TRA and TPB as a foundation, we have seen that many modifications and additions have been suggested recently to better explain action. In this final section, we provide an integrative perspective on consumer action.

First, we discuss the idea of **anticipated emotions**, which combines elements of cognition with affect. Next, we present the model of goal-directed behaviour, which combines anticipated emotions with the variables under the TPB and some of the new variables and processes discussed earlier in this chapter. Finally, we propose a comprehensive framework that incorporates most of the new ideas considered herein. The framework has some similarity to Prochaska and Di Clemente's (1984) transtheoretical approach, in that it proposes different stages of self-regulation (see also Bagozzi 1992; Prochaska et al. 1992).

Anticipated emotions

Consideration of anticipated emotions (AEs) in decision making is a relatively recent topic. Anticipated regret was an early emotion studied in this regard by Kahneman and Tversky (1982) in their 'simulation heuristic'. More recently, a number of social psychologists have expanded on AEs and performed empirical tests. Parker et al. (1995) found that anticipated negative affect influenced the intention to commit driving violations. Richard et al. (1995) found that anticipated affective reactions toward performance of safe sexual behaviours significantly predicted intentions to perform these practices (see also Sutton et al. 1999). Their study was limited to negative emotions measured with three items: worried–not worried, regret–no regret and tense–relaxed. Sheeran and Orbell (1999a) discovered that anticipated regret affected intentions to play the lottery.

A somewhat different perspective on AEs was taken by Bagozzi et al. (1998) who proposed that both anticipated positive and negative emotions are relevant to goal-directed behaviour. Frijda (1993: 393) noted that 'little systematic research exists on the actual relationships between emotions and corresponding changes in . . . goal-directed behaviors'. Bagozzi et al. (1998) built their approach on two frameworks: Oatley and Johnson-Laird's (1987) communicative theory (see also Oatley 1992; and discussion in Chapter 5) and Stein and colleagues' theory of emotion episodes (for example Stein et al. 1996).

Oatley and Johnson-Laird (1987) propose that a major function of emotions is to assist organisms with limited resources in the management of multiple goals in an uncertain world. Emotions are evoked (Oatley and Johnson-Laird 1987: 35): 'at a significant juncture of a plan . . . typically . . . when the evaluation (conscious or unconscious) of the likely success of a plan changes', and the function of emotions is to communicate to the cognitive system or to other people (in the case of mutual plans) which part of the goal structure requires attention. Positive (euphoric) emotions are associated with the attainment of a (sub)goal, which usually leads to a decision to continue with the current plan, whereas negative (dysphoric) emotions result from problems with ongoing plans and failures to achieve desired goals. Such interruptions then lead to problem-solving activities in which existing goal structures are revised and new plans aimed at dealing with the problem are developed.

A conceptually similar approach is taken by Stein and her associates (for example Stein et al. 1993, 1996). She proposed that changes in the status of valued goals lead to emotional experiences that then evoke goal-directed behaviour aimed at maintaining or reaching desired outcomes, or avoiding or escaping from undesired outcomes. Specifically, the process starts with the occurrence of a precipitating event which, if attended to, is appraised in terms of whether or not it is relevant to the pursuit of valued goals (in the sense of facilitating or obstructing goal attainment) and whether it makes goal success or goal failure more or less certain. Different emotions arise as a result of different appraisals. For example, an event that establishes the certainty of goal success will lead to happiness, whereas an event that signals certain goal failure, coupled with a belief that the valued goal cannot be reinstated, will evoke sadness. Depending on the nature of the precipitating event and the type of emotion experienced, a goal is generated to maintain or change the current state. Then, planning and problem-solving processes are initiated, and if an acceptable plan becomes available this plan is enacted. Finally, the outcomes of goal-directed behaviour are monitored. The process is dynamic in that new precipitating events can initiate another cycle of emotional experiences which then lead to planning processes in a continuous goal-action-outcome sequence.

Frijda (1986, 1993) has also dealt extensively with the relationship between emotions and behaviour. He has been a major proponent of the view that the experience of emotions involves an awareness of action readiness and that different emotions are associated with characteristic action tendencies. Modes of action readiness include moving toward, moving away, attending, rejecting, showing disinterest, moving against, and interrupting an activity. In a series of studies Frijda (1987; Frijda et al. 1989) has shown that emotions can be described in terms of both situational appraisals and modes of action readiness. For example, fear is associated with avoidance and it is induced by uncontrollable events about which one is uncertain whether one can cope (Frijda 1987). Frijda et al. (1989: 213) conclude that '[e]vents are appraised as emotionally relevant when they appear to favour or harm the individual's concerns: his/her major goals, motives, or sensitivities' and that 'different states of action readiness are elicited by different appraisals'. Frijda (1986: 98) specifically argues that emotions are often defined by an intentional structure and that these intentional structures are 'engendered as part of the plan to fulfil a given action tendency'. Furthermore, although he does not discuss the issue in detail, Frijda (1986: 97) acknowledges the possibility that behaviour 'can be motivated by the anticipation of emotion that could or will occur,' and this idea will be an important component of our own framework to be discussed next (see also Carver and Scheier 1998).

With this as background, Bagozzi et al. (1998) proposed that 17 AEs (7 positive: excited, delighted, happy, glad, satisfied, proud, self-assured; 10 negative: angry, frustrated, guilt, ashamed, sad, disappointed, depressed, worried, uncomfortable, fearful) function to influence volitions in decision making.

The 17 emotions were found to form separate positive and negative factors acting as independent variables, but the authors left open the possibility that multiple, distinct positive and multiple, distinct negative factors can exist, depending on the appraisals people make of anticipated goal attainment and goal failure. Many goals involve positive and negative consequences in these senses. For a different approach that applies to the case where products have attributes in conflict, see Luce (1998) who studied choices where avoidance options were and were not available.

A key hypothesis governing the effects of AEs is the following (Bagozzi et al. 1998). A decision maker must be capable of 'imagining the possible' (that is, identifying and appraising the consequences occurring if one were to achieve one's goal *and* fail to achieve one's goal). The thought processes entail a type of forward-looking counterfactual thinking (see presentation below). The decision maker generates alternative consequences to imagined goal success and goal failure, which then serve as input for appraisals and the generation of anticipated emotional responses. By imagining what would happen if one failed to achieve a personal goal, a decision maker elaborates upon the goal situation and sets the stage for emotional appraisals. Note appraisals need not be, and often are not, deliberative but can be automatic.

Bagozzi et al. (1998) verified the effects of AEs in a study of 406 adult consumers trying to regulate their body weight. It was found that (a) positive and negative AEs influenced dieting and exercising volitions (that is, intentions, plans and anticipated expenditure of effort), (b) volitions determined dieting and exercising goal-directed behaviours, (c) these, in turn, impacted goal attainment/failure over the period of the upcoming month, and (d) goal attainment/failure fed back on positive and negative goal-outcome emotions.

An important issue in Bagozzi et al.'s (1998) theory of AEs is how forward-looking counterfactuals function. Quite a bit of research has been performed on counterfactual thinking in recent years (for example Roese and Olson 1995). Gleicher et al. (1995: 294) call forward-looking counterfactuals, **prefactuals** (see also Boninger et al. 1994a; Strathman et al. 1994).

Gleicher et al. (1995: 284) suggest that 'individuals may think about imaginary alternatives to events in terms of the implications of these events for the future . . . People's . . . behavior . . . may very well be determined by what the counterfactuals imply for the future'. Two mechanisms were hypothesized by Gleicher et al. (1995) for serving as the basis by which counterfactuals operate to influence intentions and behaviour:

First, when a person generates a counterfactual that reverses a negative outcome, he or she is likely to make the attribution that there is an effective action that can be taken in the future . . . [Second] when an individual thinks about a counterfactual in advance, the motivation to avoid this negative affect influences behavioral choices.

(Gleicher et al. 1995: 294–5)

Two studies supported the above role for prefactuals in decision making. Boninger et al. (1994b) found that prefactuals with regard to the purchase of insurance in a laboratory game influenced subsequent action to take insurance. Likewise, Gleicher et al. (1994) found that prefactuals concerning condom use affected positive attitudes; however, intentions to use condoms were not influenced by prefactuals, although the difference in means between experimental and control groups were in the predicted direction.

We propose that people anticipate the implications of acting by forming prefactual emotions toward the consequences of achieving and not achieving a person goal. Following Roese and Olson (1995: 21), we assume that the motivational basis for prefactual thinking lies in the assessment of the alternatives in terms of one's personal welfare. That is, negative outcomes and experiences are aversive, so people should be motivated to avoid them; positive outcomes and experiences are rewarding, so people should be motivated to approach them.

A question that can be raised about attempts to introduce AEs into the TPB and similar models is whether the conceptualization of AEs and its measures overlap with A_{act} and its measures (Perugini and Bagozzi 2001a). The theoretical specification and empirical measurement of AEs differ fundamentally from the specification and measurement of both A_{act} and AEs as proposed heretofore. Consider first A_{act}. Attitude is conceived as 'a psychological tendency that is expressed by evaluating a particular entity with some degree of favour or disfavour' (Eagly and Chaiken 1993: 1, emphasis in original removed). Under the TRA and TPB, A_{act} is formulated to refer to a target behaviour and is measured by such bipolar semantic differential items as good–bad, harmful–beneficial, rewarding–punishing and unpleasant–pleasant. The psychological tendency embodied by an attitude is sometimes termed an acquired behavioural disposition (Campbell 1963). Acquisition of an attitude is thought to be primarily via learning.

The nature and role of AEs differ from that entailed by A_{act} in attitude theories in three main respects, and concern the referent, underlying process, and measurement of attitudes, respectively. First, A_{act} under the TRA and TPB focuses upon what one does or can do, whereas AEs focus, not upon action, but rather upon achievement of personal goals. Previously, researchers have taken one approach or the other. Under the TRA and TPB, actions are the referents for all antecedents. The approach taken by Bagozzi et al. (1998) rests on the argument that people, when deliberating to act or not in goal-directed situations, take into account the emotional consequences of both achieving and not achieving a sought for goal. The approaches to AEs taken by Parker et al. (1995), Richard et al. (1995), Sheeran and Orbell (1999a) and Sutton et al. (1999) focus primarily on negative affect alone and seem to conceive of these as attitudes.

A second difference between the approach taken by Bagozzi et al. (1998) and the TPB and related models, beyond divergence in referents, concerns the theoretical processes underlying the effects of A_{act} versus AEs. As a disposition to respond in a favourable or unfavourable manner, A_{act} arises through learning, whereby a person acquires a reaction to an object or action over a period of time or through repeated contact accompanied by reinforcement. An attitude is an evaluative response toward an object or act that, once learned, is triggered automatically when one is exposed to the object or act or thinks about it (Fazio 1995). By contrast, the processes behind the functioning of AEs are more dynamic and entail self-regulation in response to feedback (Bagozzi 1992; Carver and Scheier 1998). That is, one first has a goal, then appraises the consequences of achieving and not achieving that goal, with corresponding positive and negative emotions arising. An attitude is typically constant over reasonable periods of time and is not formulated as a response contingent on the occurrence of particular happenings to be appraised. The proposed functioning of AEs are, in contrast, specifically contingent on one's appraisal of goal achievement/goal failure, which changes from time to time, depending on the context. An implicit comparison is made between one's goal as a standard or reference value and achieving and failing to achieve that goal, with anticipated emotions as consequences. Attitudes do not function in this manner but are more disposition-like responses to a fixed object or act.

A third distinction we wish to make between A_{act} and AEs occurs at the level of measurement. When people are asked to respond with their attitudes, they are forced to make a choice of favourability *or* unfavourability. This is a consequence of the common practice of using bipolar items to indicate respondents' attitudes. By contrast, for the measurement of AEs, we argue that it is important to use unipolar items (for example the experience of excitement along a 'not at all' to 'very much' continuum). In a study of affect, Bagozzi et al. (1999b) found that positive and negative affect can be positively or negatively related (or unrelated) to each other, depending on the circumstances. This finding is in line with related evidence for basic differences between positive and negative emotional reactions (see Chapter 3). To use a bipolar scale to measure emotions (as is done in attitude theory) would make positive and negative affect mutually exclusive by definition and not permit respondents the opportunity to express their differential relevance. Previous research found that positive and negative AEs were positively correlated yet clearly differentiated ($\phi = 0.50$; Bagozzi et al. 1998).

In sum, one type of revision to the TPB and similar models proposed herein adds AEs as parallel predictors along with the traditional independent variables found in the models. Whereas the TPB specifies that action is the target referent of all independent variables, defines A_{act} as a disposition-like tendency to respond favourably or unfavourably toward the action, and uses bipolar items to measure A_{act}, the theory proposed by Bagozzi et al. (1998) stipulates that the referents of AEs are personal goals, AEs function as independent variables based upon a decision process that takes into account judged consequences of goal achievement and goal failure, and AEs are measured as unipolar reactions.

The model of goal-directed behaviour

Perugini and Bagozzi (2001a) combined AEs with desires and frequency and recency effects of past behaviour, along with the variables from the TPB, to produce an integrative approach known as the model of goal-directed behaviour (MGB). Figure 4.4 presents the MGB, where it can be seen that (a) A_{act}, positive and negative AEs (that is, PAE and NAE), SN, PBC and frequency of past behaviour (FPB) are direct determinants of desires (D), (b) D, PBC and FPB influence I, and (c) action (A) is a function of FPB, I, PBC and recency of past behaviour (RPB). The MGB broadens and deepens the TPB by incorporating a number of important advances found in recent research.

The MGB was tested in two surveys: one a study of dieting and exercising as means to body weight regulation goals, and the second an investigation of studying goals (Perugini and Bagozzi 2001a). In both studies, desires mediated the influences of antecedents on intentions, and intentions influenced action, as shown in Figure 4.4. For exercising and dieting, PAE, SN and FPB were significant determinants of D, while PBC influenced A for exercising but not dieting. Likewise, FPB influenced I and RPB influenced A for both exercising and dieting, but PBC influenced A for exercising but not dieting. For studying, A_{act}, NAE, SN, PBC and FPB influenced D, and FPB influenced A; FPB influenced A, but neither PBC nor RPB affected A.

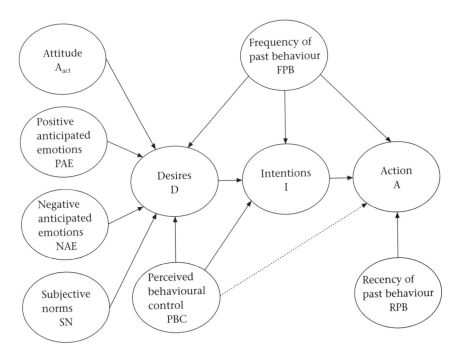

Figure 4.4 The model of goal-directed behaviour

A comparison to the TPB showed the following. Under the TPB, explained variance of I was 0.58 and 0.34 for exercising and dieting, respectively, and explained variance of A was 0.38 and 0.19 for exercising and dieting, respectively. This can be compared to explained variance under the MGB, where it was found that the respective values for I were 0.78 and 0.74 and the respective values for A were 0.46 and 0.25. Likewise, under the TPB, explained variance of I was 0.34 and A 0.15 for studying. By comparison, under the MGB, the respective values were 0.53 and 0.24.

In sum, significantly more variance in I and A was accounted for by the MGB than the TPB. Equally important, the MGB provides greater understanding of how I and A are produced. An important finding was that D provides sufficient impetus for I formation and channels the effects of the antecedents. The role of anticipated emotions is an important new antecedent. The MGB not only accounts for more variation in I and A than the TPB but also provides a richer explanation for how these variables arise.

Perugini and Conner (2000) extended the MGB by adding goal desires as a predictor of behavioural desires and adding goal perceived feasibility as a predictor of PBC. In their study of intention formation, they found that the explained variance in intentions due to the TPB, MGB, and the extended MGB yielded respective values of 0.30, 0.74 and 0.76, demonstrating the superiority of the MGB over the TPB. Also PAE proved again to be important antecedents.

A comprehensive framework for studying consumer action

Given the many advances in attitude theory in recent years, we wish to provide a comprehensive framework summarizing many of these developments. Figure 4.5 shows our integrative framework of consumer action (see also Bagozzi 2000b). As we have already discussed many of the variables and linkages in this figure, we shall focus on the facets not considered yet.

One of the least studied, but most intriguing, aspects of action is the functioning of non-conscious processes very early in the decision process. We have labelled this 'unconscious cerebral initiative and the **somatic marker hypothesis**' in Figure 4.5, and here is how these processes are believed to work. Libet (1993) discovered that people's conscious decisions to initiate bodily movements in choice situations occurs, as expected, before the movement occurs (about 200 milliseconds before) but happens, unexpectedly, *after* the onset of the readiness potential which is involved in sending a signal to the muscles to move. The readiness potential occurs about 500 milliseconds before the movement and 300 milliseconds before the conscious decision. It seems that unconscious processes initiate decisions *before* the choice is made to do so. Libet explains this by positing that decision makers have the ability to 'veto' or stop a bodily movement in the early

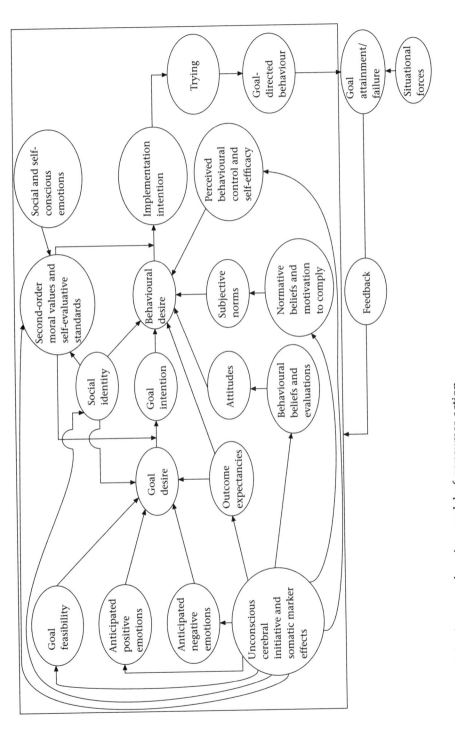

Figure 4.5 A comprehensive model of consumer action

process of initiation, even after making a conscious choice. In other words, decision makers exercise control over their actions by choosing to allow the action to go ahead or not, after the action has been unconsciously initiated.

Damasio (1994, 1999) offers a somewhat different account of how non-conscious emotions affect decision making. He maintains that prior to the processing of pros and cons characteristic of rational decision making, people experience pleasant or unpleasant feelings which highlight options and create either positive or negative biases, which favour or eliminate options from consideration (Damasio 1994: 173–4). Damasio termed this the 'somatic-marker hypothesis'. We suggest that such unconscious processes influence or bias a number of antecedents to decision making. As shown in Figure 4.5, desirability and feasibility of goals, beliefs and expectations, normative beliefs and motivation to comply, anticipated emotions, and moral and non-moral values are directly connected to such unconscious processes.

We might speculate that declarative knowledge processed rationally by consumers (with regard to facts, alternative goals and products, consequences of consumption, and various expectations) is influenced by non-conscious preference biases residing in the brain and arising from previous emotional experience associated with similar decision problems. Bechara et al. (1997) present research showing that such covert processes bias decision making prior to cognitive evaluation and reasoning and without awareness occurring on the part of decision makers. The authors suggested that the non-conscious processes guide or shape behaviour, before conscious processing commences, and function to produce better decisions, especially to the extent that learning accumulates as a consequence of previous rewards and punishments, which become stored as non-declarative dispositional knowledge. Bargh and Barndollar (1996) give yet another perspective on unconscious influences on action.

Figure 4.5 also shows that moral values and self-evaluative standards regulate consumer desires. Values are 'the criteria people use to select and justify actions and to evaluate people (including the self) and events' (Schwartz 1992: 1). Values are normative concepts and address questions of right and wrong and prescriptions for acting. Very little work has been done with moral values, per se, in consumer research, but we feel that they can be influential determinants in decision making. Group norms held by individual consumers might also be considered a type of value. In Carver and Scheier's (1998) cybernetic theory of control, values function as abstract standards that constrain programme goals. Self-evaluative standards concern who a person is and desires to be. Along with moral values they function as second-order mental states to regulate both goal selection and goal striving (see Figure 4.5).

Bagozzi and Lee (2001a) investigated three sources of social influence in attitude theory: compliance, internalization and identification. Compliance is a type of interpersonal influence where the complier desires to gain favourable reactions from significant others (for example social approval, liking, praise) and/or to deter unfavourable reactions from significant others (for example social rejection, disapproval, displeasure). Subjective norms capture compliance processes in this sense.

Internalization processes can be represented through the effects of group norms and might be considered a special case of values. Social influence due to group norms is reflected in shared values or goals as perceived by a decision maker between themself and members of a group to which they belong. To the extent that one's values or goals are congruent with those of members of one's reference group, we would expect that one's desire to act in accordance with group norms will increase.

Liska (1984: 63) points out that the TRA was formulated to explain volitional behaviours of a personal sort and not behaviours dependent on 'the cooperation of others'. The many successes in the literature finding that intentions predict behaviour have occurred when both variables include personal referents in their formulations: personal intentions predict personal behaviours. Likewise, the explanation of intentions works best when its antecedents are formulated with common referents. We would expect, for example, personal attitudes to predict personal intentions well but not necessarily group intentions. Similarly, group variables should not necessarily explain personal intentions as main effects. Indeed, in Terry and Hogg's (1996) research, an inspection of their correlation tables reveals that the correlation between group identification and personal intentions was $r = 15$ (ns) in Study 1 and $r = -0.04$ (ns) in Study 2. Likewise, research explaining personal intentions on the basis of self-identity finds that only about 1 per cent of additional variance is accounted for by this variable (see meta-analysis in Conner and Armitage 1998: 1446).

We hypothesize in Figure 4.5 that *social-identity* influences desire and intentions. Our rationale draws upon **social identity** and social categorization theories (for example Tajfel 1981; Turner 1985; Hogg and Abrams 1988; Terry et al. 1999). Tajfel (1978) suggested that a person achieves a social identity through self-awareness of one's membership in a group and the emotional and evaluative significance of this membership. Building on these insights, Ellemers et al. (1999: 372) proposed that three components comprise one's social identity: 'a *cognitive* component (a cognitive awareness of one's membership in a social group – self-categorisation), an *evaluative* component (a positive and negative value connotation attached to this group membership – group self-esteem), and an *emotional* component (a sense of emotional involvement with the group – **affective commitment**)'. Construct validity for the measures of these components of social identity has been demonstrated by Bergami and Bagozzi (2000) and Ellemers et al. (1999).

Social identities prescribe and instigate behaviours for the benefit of group members. Ellemers et al. (1999) studied experimentally formed groups and found that aspects of social identity influenced in-group favouritism (in terms of evaluative ratings and outcome allocations). Similarly, Bergami and Bagozzi (2000) found in an investigation of organization employees that social identity influenced organization citizenship behaviours (a form of in-group favouritism).

Support for the influence of social identity can be found in Bagozzi and Lee's (2001, 2002) study of restaurant patronage by friendship groups. Similarly, Dholakia and Bagozzi (2001) found, in their study of people in collaborative browsing and virtual community internet groups, that social identity was a key factor in decision making.

In conclusion, we have come a long way from the simple TRA and TPB models. The TRA and TPB have been shown to omit consideration of important variables and processes. One class of omissions occurs as antecedents to attitudes, subjective norms and other reasons for acting. The theories have been shown as well to neglect processes of decision making with respect to goal setting. An important variable in this regard is desire – both the desire for a goal and the desire to form an implementation intention or perform a goal-directed behaviour. The need for desire arises because the multiple reasons for acting must be integrated and motivation must be provided for decision making. Contemporary theories also neglect to consider the role played in decision making of moral behaviour and self-evaluative guidelines, which we propose function as second-order variables and regulate desire. Finally, a major oversight of the TRA and TPB is the failure to consider post-intention processes. Here the set of mental and physical activities comprising trying need to be considered in order to explain how decision making influences goal attainment/failure. Trying encompasses the initiation of goal-directed behaviours, monitoring of progress in goal pursuit, regulating various control and guidance processes, overcoming impediments, resisting temptation, re-evaluating one's goal and plans, if necessary, and maintaining commitment. Self-regulation thus involves cognitive ('cool') as well as emotional ('hot') processes that are interrelated (for example Metcalfe and Mischel 1999). The study of consumer behaviour provides many exciting opportunities for researchers and challenges for marketers and change agents, as we move toward consideration of how cognitive, emotional, social and moral processes shape consumer action.

Suggested readings

Ajzen, I. (1991) The theory of planned behavior, *Organizational Behavior and Human Decision Processes*, 50: 179–211. An extended development of the theory of planned behaviour and review of empirical research.

Ajzen, I. and Fishbein, M. (1980) *Understanding Attitudes and Predicting Social Behavior.* Englewood Cliffs, NJ: Prentice-Hall. An update of ideas presented in Fishbein and Ajzen (1975) with a number of chapters exploring the theory of reasoned action in applied settings.

Bagozzi, R.P. (2000a) On the concept of intentional social action in consumer behavior, *Journal of Consumer Research*, 27: 388–96. Introduces the concept of shared or 'we' intentions and how they relate to social action.

Bagozzi, R.P. (2000b) The poverty of economic explanations of consumption and an action theory alternative, *Managerial and Decision Economics*, 21: 95–109. Presents a comprehensive model of consumer action and its determinants and contrasts it with economic theory. The model integrates attitudes, cognitive processes, desire, emotion and volition as explanatory concepts.

Bagozzi, R.P. and Dholakia, U. (1999) Goal-setting and goal-striving in consumer behavior, *Journal of Marketing*, 63: 19–32. Reviews the literature on goal-setting and goal pursuit from multiple research traditions and relates these to consumer research.

Carver, C.S. and Scheier, M.F. (1998) *On the Self-Regulation of Behavior*. Cambridge: Cambridge University Press. The latest presentation of the authors' cybernetic theory of control and its relation to self-regulation.

Gollwitzer, P.M. and Bargh, J.A. (1996) *The Psychology of Action: Linking Cognition and Motivation to Behavior*. New York: Guilford. A collection of chapters by leading psychologists into goals, schemas, planning and other allied areas from social psychology. See esp. pp. 287–312.

Perugini, M. and Bagozzi, R.P. (2001a) The role of desires and anticipated emotions in goal-directed behaviours: broadening and deepening the theory of planned behaviour, *British Journal of Social Psychology*, 40: 79–98. Integrates the concepts of anticipated emotions, desires, and recency and frequency of past behaviour with the theory of planned behaviour and presents empirical tests of the model.

5

Attitude change: the elaboration likelihood model of persuasion

One of the most important aspects of attitudes is their presumed influence on subsequent behaviour. Attitudes have been conceptualized as an important mediator of behaviour (Allport 1935; Fishbein and Ajzen 1975; Ajzen and Fishbein 1977, 1980; Fazio et al. 1983; Fazio and Williams 1986; Petty and Cacioppo 1986; Fazio et al. 1989; Fazio 1995; Petty et al. 1995b). For example, if you have a positive attitude towards the practice of safe sex, you are more likely to behave in a manner consistent with safe sex practices. You might be more likely to use a condom, refrain from casual sex with strangers, or perhaps abstain from sex altogether.

Given this presumed influence of attitudes on behaviour, attitudes have been viewed as an important means by which to modify or change behaviour. If I want you to reduce your unsafe sex practices, one cogent way for me to accomplish this goal is to change your attitude such that it is more positive towards safe sex behaviours. Similarly, if I want you to purchase my product, the probability of such a purchase should increase if I can change your attitude to be more favourable toward my product. As such, persuasion (that is, attitude change) has been viewed as a key to behavioural change.

These examples raise two fundamental issues. First, when do attitudes actually guide behaviour? If I am able to change your attitude towards safe sex, does that insure that you will use a condom in the future? Second, how does one go about changing a person's attitude? Although the primary focus of this chapter will be on the latter question, it will become apparent by the end of the chapter that in fact the two questions are closely related. An understanding of the psychological processes by which attitudes are changed provides insight into when (and how) attitudes are likely to guide behaviour.

A short history of persuasion

Not surprisingly, persuasion has been of interest to people from time in memorial. Aristotle sought to explicate the laws of persuasion in his classic text *Rhetoric*. The ancient Romans, in the time of Cicero, as well as the Italians during the Renaissance, also attempted to understand the principles underlying persuasion (see McGuire 1969). Clearly, these early approaches relied on philosophic and introspective insight rather than on empirical approaches. What is noteworthy, however, is that the question of how attitudes are changed has been of keen interest to humankind since the earliest of our writings.

Early empirical investigations of persuasion

One of the earliest attempts to experimentally investigate the effects of persuasion over time was conducted by Peterson and Thurstone (1933, 1970).[1] Peterson and Thurstone exposed junior high and high school children in different cities to different films. These films were designed to change specific attitudes (for example attitudes towards individuals of different nationalities and races, attitudes towards war, and attitudes toward different types of punishment).

The attitudes targeted by the films were measured both immediately after the children had seen the film, and then again from 2 to 19 months later. Four of the films exhibited the hypothesized pattern of **attitude decay**: the attitudes were most influenced immediately following exposure to the film and this influence dissipated over time. However, one of the films exhibited a most unexpected pattern. The attitudes of the students who saw the film *Four Sons* were even more favourable toward the attitude object (people of German nationality) after six months than they were immediately after viewing the film. That is, the attitudes became more, rather than less, influenced by the persuasive merits of the film over time. These surprising findings were harbingers of often confusing and seemingly contradictory research findings to come.

Hovland-Yale Communication and Persuasion Research Program

Although psychologists studied persuasion throughout the early and mid-1900s, it was the work of Carl Hovland and his colleagues (for example Hovland et al. 1953; Hovland 1957) that provided the first programmatic and experimental approach to understanding the persuasion process. The Hovland-Yale Communication and Persuasion (HYCP) group sought to apply fundamental principles derived from research on learning to the phenomenon of persuasion. They hypothesized that the basic processes underlying persuasion are *attention, comprehension, yielding* and *retention* (which were conceptualized as four necessary stages for persuasion to occur). They hypothesized that it is necessary that an individual attend to the persuasive information, comprehend that information, yield to the information and then retain the information over time. Note, however, that this perspective predicts that these are independent stages. Thus, although you may pay attention to an advertisement, this does not insure that you will comprehend the advertisement. Similarly, attention and comprehension do not imply that you will necessarily yield to the advertisement. And even if you do yield, there is no guarantee that you will retain the information from the advertisement (McGuire 1989).

In a programme of research that spanned from the late 1940s to the early 1960s (and can be said to continue to this day with the theoretical perspective advanced by McGuire 1985, 1989), Hovland and colleagues explored how different variables influence this process. The HYCP group classified the persuasion variables according to four categories: *source, message, recipient* and *channel* factors (see Petty and Cacioppo (1981) for a detailed discussion of the research group). The HYCP group conducted a vast stream of research that sought to understand how persuasion variables influence the process variables (for example Hovland et al. 1949; Hovland 1951; Hovland et al. 1953; Hovland 1957; Hovland and Janis 1959; Hovland and Rosenberg 1960; Sherif and Hovland 1961).

Although the HYCP provided a useful approach, it was not without its limitations (see Petty et al. 2002). Perhaps the greatest difficulty with this approach was that its most basic tenet, that learning of the persuasive information underlies attitude change and persistence, failed to receive consistent empirical support.

Specifically, the HYCP group hypothesized that it was the comprehension and learning of persuasive information that guided attitude change and it was the ability to remember the persuasive information that accounted for **attitude persistence**. Little empirical evidence, however, supported the view that message learning is a necessary or even sufficient step (Greenwald 1968; Petty and Cacioppo 1981; McGuire 1985). Perhaps of greatest concern, the influence of memory for the persuasive information on attitudes, both immediately following exposure to persuasive information and over time, was weak at best (see Greenwald 1968). These findings suggest that the ability to remember persuasive information does not mediate attitude change or persistence. Instead, the evidence suggested that message comprehension and learning can occur without attitude change, and that an individual's attitudes can change without learning the specific information in the communication. This contradiction provided the basis for an approach to persuasion to arise in the late 1960s and early 1970s and is presented shortly, the **cognitive response approach**.

Balance process theories of persuasion

An approach to persuasion, distinct from that offered by the HYCP group, emerged in the late 1950s and flourished throughout the 1960s. The approach was based upon the notion that individuals prefer consistency (that is, balance) in their own attitudes, thoughts, and behaviours (that is, intrapersonal balance) as well as their interpersonal relationships (that is, interpersonal balance). As a consequence, individuals are motivated to change their attitudes such that they are consistent with their own behaviour (for example Festinger 1957; Festinger and Carlsmith 1959) and such that they agree with their friends and disagree with their enemies (for example Heider 1958; Insko 1984). From the perspective of these approaches, individuals are motivated to maintain both intrapersonal and interpersonal balance, and attitudes often are changed in order to satisfy this basic motivation.[2]

This approach to persuasion won over researchers in the 1960s (for example Abelson et al. 1968; cf. Greenwald et al. 1968; see Petty and Cacioppo 1981 for a review). However, tensions between the theories began to emerge concerning the processes by which balance was motivated. Specifically, **cognitive dissonance** hypothesized that attitudes were changed in order to reduce internal feelings of discomfort that arose in response to becoming aware of inconsistencies (Festinger 1957; Festinger and Carlsmith 1959), whereas **self-perception** theory hypothesized that individuals merely inferred their attitudes from their own behaviour and that internal feelings of discomfort were not necessary to explain balance motivation (Bem 1972). This theoretical tension led to a stream of research designed to demonstrate which process was correct (for example Greenwald 1975; Kiesler and Munson 1975).

Fazio et al. (1977) provided a resolution to this debate. Rather than showing *which* theory was correct, Fazio et al. (1977) demonstrated *when* each theory was correct. Specifically, Fazio et al. (1977) provided evidence that the extent of the discrepant information (for example one's own behaviour) moderated which process accounted for the attitude change. When the discrepant behaviour is extremely different from one's attitude, that is, outside of one's latitude of acceptance (M. Sherif and Hovland 1961; C.W. Sherif et al. 1965), internal feelings of discomfort mediate attitude change. When the discrepant behaviour is not extremely different (that is, inside of one's latitude of acceptance), self-perception mediates attitude change. What is noteworthy about this resolution is that it foreshadows a key construct of the Elaboration Likelihood Model. Variables (such as attitude-discrepant behaviour) can influence persuasion by different, specifiable processes.

Cognitive response approach

The cognitive response (CR) approach (Greenwald 1968; Petty et al. 1981b) was developed in part to provide an alternative theory of persuasion that resolved the empirical inconsistencies that underlay the HYCP approach. Recall that studies consistently revealed a low correlation between learning of the persuasive information and persuasion. The CR approach hypothesized that these low correlations were indicative of the fact that message learning does not mediate attitude change. Instead, the CR approach advanced the proposition that the impact of variables on persuasion depends on the extent to which individuals generate and consider their own idiosyncratic thoughts to the information presented. Basically, the CR approach posits that individuals are active participants in the persuasion process. As such, they attempt to relate message elements to their existing bases of knowledge. And it is the thoughts that are self-generated as a result of this active participation that mediate attitude change. As such, attitude change and persistence should be mediated by cognitive responses, rather than message learning. Research emerged demonstrating that, under certain conditions, strong correlations did emerge between cognitive responses and attitude change, as well as cognitive responses and attitude persistence (for example Greenwald 1968; Petty 1977).

The conflicting findings of persuasion research

The field of persuasion was both blessed and cursed by the shear quantity of research conducted throughout the 1950s, 1960s and 1970s. What were particularly troubling were the inconsistent findings often uncovered. One set of research findings would suggest that a variable increased persuasion. Another set would suggest that the same variable decreased persuasion. And yet another set would suggest that the same variable did not influence persuasion at all! To illustrate, consider the variable, source **trustworthiness**. What could be more obvious than the prediction that trustworthy sources should engender more persuasion than untrustworthy sources? Hovland et al. (1953) hypothesized that an endorser associated with high trustworthiness engenders greater message acceptance than an endorser associated with moderate or low trustworthiness. And it is the message acceptance that is hypothesized to mediate attitude change. It is possible to derive the similar predictions from the **balance process** theories of persuasion. For example, one should be motivated to agree more with trustworthy than untrustworthy sources.

A series of studies were conducted in order to examine this seemingly obvious prediction. Hovland et al. (1953), for example, report the findings from several studies that examined the influence of source credibility on persuasion. In these studies, credibility is defined as the combination of a source's expertise (that is, does the source have knowledge on the topic) and trustworthiness (that is, can the source be trusted to provide accurate information). As predicted, high rather than low, source credibility was found to generally lead to greater persuasion. For example, Hovland and Weiss (1951) gave people different messages associated with either high or low credible sources. Collapsed across topics, the high credible sources were more persuasive overall. However, examination of the specific message-source combinations revealed a potentially important boundary condition to this result. Namely, the positive influence of source credibility on persuasion was stronger for the topics Atomic Submarines and Steel Shortage than for the topics Antihistamines and Future of Movies. In fact, for the topic Future of Movies, the low credible source produced somewhat more attitude change than the high credible source.

This apparent confusion as to a source's influence on persuasion is even greater when the more specific construct of trustworthiness rather than the more general construct of credibility is examined. In one study, Kelman and Hovland (1953) sought to examine how perceived trustworthiness of a source influences attitude change. People were told that a message either was from a source who would benefit were the advocacy adopted (that is, the source possessed self-interest in the topic) or that the source would not benefit regardless of the outcome. Although the source manipulation was able to produce differences in how trustworthy the participants perceived the sources to be, there was no difference in the persuasion resulting from the sources. That is, sources of high and low trustworthiness produced similar amounts of attitude change. Or in other words and did not appear to influence persuasion.

To summarize, the literature suggested that sometimes trustworthiness led to greater persuasion, sometimes trustworthiness led to less persuasion, and sometimes trustworthiness did not influence persuasion at all! These confusing findings were not unique to trustworthiness. Similar findings for other variables emerged over time (for example mood: see Petty et al. 1988, 1991) and by the 1970s the field of persuasion was oft characterized (for example Kiesler and Munson 1975; Jaspers 1978; Fishbein and Ajzen 1981) as replete with conflicting empirical findings and lacking any coherent, unifying theory.

The Elaboration Likelihood Model of persuasion (ELM)

The introduction of the ELM (Petty 1977; Petty and Cacioppo 1981, 1986) provided such a coherent, unifying theory. An examination of the persuasion theories advanced through the 1970s reveals that all share the similarity of offering *a* process by which attitudes are changed. The process hypothesized to guide persuasion differs, albeit, for each theory. The HYCP approach hypothesized that attitudes are changed by the learning of persuasion information (that is, attention, comprehension, yielding and retention). Balance process theories hypothesized that attitudes are changed by motivation to maintain either intrapersonal or interpersonal consistency processes. The CR approach hypothesized that attitudes are changed as a result of the idiosyncratic thoughts and feelings that people have in response to persuasive information. Thus, all theories can be conceptualized as providing a psychological process by which attitudes are changed.

In stark theoretical contrast to these prior conceptualizations, the ELM hypothesizes that attitudes can be changed as a result of *different psychological processes* (for a discussion of the different theoretical frameworks associated with persuasion theories, see Petty 1994, 1997). The ELM groups the various processes by which attitudes can be changed into two conceptually distinct processes: those processes in which attitudes are changed as a result of effortful elaboration (often referred to as the **central route**) versus those processes in which attitudes are changed as a result of relatively non-thoughtful

Table 5.1   The postulates of the Elaboration Likelihood Model (ELM)

---

1 People are motivated to hold correct attitudes.
2 Although people want to hold correct attitudes, the amount and nature of issue-relevant elaboration in which they are willing or able to evaluate a message vary with individual and situational factors.
3 Variables can affect the amount and direction of attitude change by (a) serving as persuasive arguments, (b) serving as peripheral cues, and/or (c) affecting the extent or direction of issue and argument elaboration.
4 Variables affecting motivation and/or ability to process a message in a relatively objective manner can do so by either enhancing or reducing argument scrutiny.
5 Variables affecting message processing in a relatively biased manner can produce either a positive (favourable) or negative (unfavourable) motivational and/or ability bias to the issue-relevant thoughts attempted.
6 As motivation and/or ability to process arguments is decreased, peripheral cues become relatively more important determinants of persuasion. Conversely, as argument scrutiny is increased, peripheral cues become relatively less important determinants of persuasion.
7 Attitude changes that result mostly from processing issue-relevant arguments (central route) will show greater temporal persistence, greater prediction of behavior, and greater resistance to counter-persuasion than attitude changes that result mostly from peripheral cues.

---

processes (often referred to as the **peripheral route**). The ELM is presented in seven postulates (Petty and Cacioppo 1986; Petty and Wegener 1998) which are presented in Table 5.1.

Two routes to persuasion

The ELM predicts that a person's *motivation* and *ability* influence which process is most likely to guide persuasion. When individuals possess both motivation and ability, they are more likely to be persuaded by thoughtful elaboration of the issue-relevant persuasive information. That is, they are likely to consider the information presented, generate thoughts and feelings in response to that information, and change their attitude as a function of these cognitive responses. Conceptually, thoughtful elaboration is most similar to the process posited by the Cognitive Response approach to persuasion (Greenwald 1968; Petty et al. 1981b). It should be recalled, however, that the cognitive response approach hypothesized that *all* persuasion is mediated by cognitive responses. The ELM, however, predicts that this effortful process of attitude change is likely to mediate persuasion primarily when individuals possess both the motivation and ability to elaborate the information.

By what process are attitudes changed when individuals do not possess both motivation and ability? The ELM posits that under these conditions attitude change is most likely to be mediated by processes that do not entail the thoughtful consideration of issue-relevant information (that is, elaboration). Instead, individuals are likely to rely on (a) less effortful scrutiny of the issue-relevant information, (b) inference processes, and/or (c) associative processes. That is, when individuals do not possess both motivation and ability, the processes which guide persuasion can differ from elaboration either quantitatively (that is, extent of thought) or qualitatively (type of thought: see Petty and Wegener 1999). Under these less thoughtful conditions, processes such as classical conditioning (Staats and Statts 1958), mere exposure (Zajonc 1968), motor processes (Cacioppo et al. 1993) and heuristic shortcuts (Chaiken 1980) influence attitude change. All of these processes have been found to be more likely to guide persuasion when individuals lack motivation and/or ability (Chaiken 1980; Cacioppo et al. 1992b, 1993; Petty et al. 1993a; Priester et al. 1996).

Assessment of elaboration

One of the key contributions of the ELM, then, is to organize persuasion processes according to whether the attitude change is the result of relatively effortful elaboration or instead relatively non-thoughtful processes. A related and oft misunderstood (see Petty et al. 1993b; Petty and Wegener 1999) advance of the ELM concerns the inference of differences in elaboration as a function of a variable of interest. Specifically, the ELM provides insight into the question of how one infers whether persuasion has come about because of relatively thoughtful or non-thoughtful processes. Although many approaches to this important question have been advanced, ranging from simple self-reports of cognitive effort (Petty et al. 1977, 1980; Harkins and Petty 1981; Cacioppo et al. 1983; Batra and Ray 1986) to physiological markers of cognitive activity (Cacioppo and Petty 1979; Cacioppo et al. 1984b, 1985), two approaches have emerged as the 'gold standards' by which to infer relative differences in elaboration – the assessment of cognitive responses and the manipulation of argument quality.

Cognitive responses
One method commonly used to infer differences in the processes underlying attitude change is the measurement of cognitive responses (Greenwald 1968; Petty et al. 1981b). In this approach, both the attitude that results from a persuasive communication and the thoughts that occurred to a message recipient during exposure to the persuasive communication are assessed. These thoughts are then used in order to infer relative differences in issue-relevant thinking (that is, elaboration). Some researchers have used the total number of cognitive responses reported as an indicator of elaboration, assuming that greater elaboration results in more cognitive responses (for example Burnkrant and Howard 1984).

Other researchers have combined positive and negative thoughts in order to arrive at an index of thought positivity. The thoughts are typically combined by subtracting negative from positive thoughts (see Cacioppo et al. 1981). This index of thought positivity can then be used as a tool by which to infer differences in elaboration. For example, differences in elaboration can be inferred if individuals exposed to strong arguments report more thought positivity and individuals exposed to weak arguments report less though positivity (for example Petty et al. 1999).

Another approach to using the index of thought positivity is to examine the influence of the thoughts on the resulting attitude. Recall that elaboration is conceptualized as the process whereby the cognitive responses lead to the changed attitude. As such, one can use differences in the influence of the thought positivity index on the changed attitude (as assessed by either correlations, for example Priester and Petty (forthcoming) or by the use of mediational analyses, for example Petty et al. 1993a) as a means of inferring differences in elaboration at the time of attitude change.

Thus, it can be seen that cognitive responses can be fruitfully used in a variety of ways in order to judge relative differences in elaboration as a function of a variable of interest. Although the cognitive response approach is widely used, it is not without criticism (see Eagly and Chaiken 1993: 293–6). Much of this criticism focuses upon the correlational nature of the approach. Specifically, researchers using the cognitive response approach often wish to make the inference that, under specific conditions, thoughts are the result of effortful elaboration during the message presentation and these thoughts to attitudes. However, given the correlational nature of this approach, it is alternatively possible that, under specific conditions, the reported attitudes lead to thoughts. For example, the variable of interest might motivate recipients to justify their attitudes in their cognitive responses (Miller and Colman 1981). This enhanced motivation to justify one's attitude would likely lead to the generation of more thoughts and thoughts that were more linked to the valence of the attitudes than when motivation to justify one's attitude was low. Thus, a problem with the cognitive response approach is that it is possible to construct explanations other than elaboration during initial message exposure to explain observed differences.

The manipulation of argument quality
In response to criticisms concerning the cognitive response approach, a *manipulation of argument quality* was introduced as an alternative means of assessing the extent of issue-relevant message elaboration (Petty et al. 1976; see Petty and Cacioppo 1986: 30–44; Petty et al. 1993b). The logic of manipulating argument quality to assess the extent of thinking is that when individuals are exposed to a message under specific conditions that foster message-based elaboration, the quality of the arguments should have a larger impact on attitudes than when elaboration is low. In short, argument quality is a metric by which to measure differences in the extent that individuals elaborate content of the message.

To illustrate, consider the variable, personal relevance. In order to use the argument quality approach, an investigator would develop one set of strong and one set of weak arguments in support of a position. This pre-testing is accomplished by asking people to thoughtfully consider and cognitively respond to various arguments. Instructed thought is used in pre-testing to ascertain that the arguments would elicit different profiles of attitudes and thoughts if the recipients were carefully scrutinizing them. Those arguments that elicit predominately positive cognitive responses are classified as strong and those that elicit predominately negative cognitive responses are classified as weak. Other features of the arguments, such as equating both strong and weak arguments for potential non-thoughtful cues are also important. For a more detailed explanation of using argument quality to assess extent of thinking, see Petty and Cacioppo (1986).

Once strong and weak arguments have been generated for a position, people are then randomly assigned to either high or low personal relevance conditions *and* to receive either strong or weak arguments, resulting in four experimental conditions. Evidence consistent with the hypothesis that variations in personal relevance are associated with different levels of issue-relevant message-based elaboration would be found in an interaction of personal relevance with argument quality. This interaction would reveal that individuals under conditions of high personal relevance show greater attitudinal differentiation for argument quality than individuals under conditions of low personal relevance. Such an interaction is graphed in Figure 5.1. That is, the greater influence of argument quality on attitudes for high rather than low personal relevance suggests that individuals who receive message associated with high personal relevance base their attitudes on a thoughtful scrutiny of the arguments more so than individuals who receive a message associated with low personal relevance (see Petty and Cacioppo 1986).

Since its introduction, argument quality has been manipulated along with a large number of variables in an attempt to examine the impact of these variables on message elaboration. This widespread adoption of the argument quality manipulation in order to assess message-based elaboration is in part due to its experimental, rather than correlational, design. Given the experimental nature of the argument quality manipulation, it is more reasonable to infer that the variable of interest is causes differences in message-based elaboration. Also, the interaction rather than main effect approach of the argument quality manipulation makes it more difficult to construct alternative explanations for the data, since these alternative explanations would need to account for the argument quality X variable of interest interaction.

Elaboration likelihood continuum

Recall that motivation and ability are hypothesized to determine which process underlies persuasion. The ELM advances the notion that these two factors

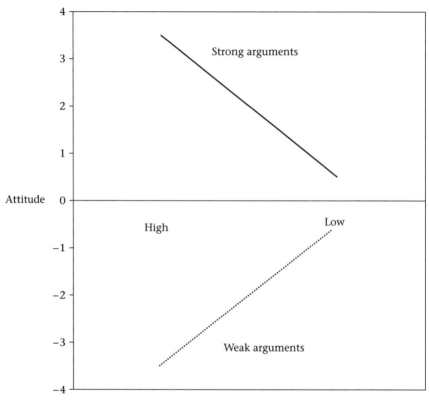

Personal relevance

Figure 5.1   The manipulation of argument quality in order to infer differences elaboration

influence the *likelihood* that an individual will *elaborate* persuasive informa-tion (that is, the elaboration likelihood). It is important to note that elabora-tion likelihood is conceptualized as a continuum, rather than as two discrete states (see Petty and Cacioppo 1986; Petty et at. 1994; Petty and Wegner 1999). As individuals move from one end of the continuum to the other, the amount of effort they expend on thoughtfully considering the issue-relevant information ranges from none at all to scrutinizing and considering all information.

The ELM assumes that across the entire range of the elaboration likelihood continuum individuals are motivated to hold accurate (that is, correct) atti-tudes (see Postulate 1). However, the effort that individuals expend in order to arrive at their attitudes is hypothesized to differ along the continuum (see Postulates 2 and 6). One important manner by which variables influence persuasion is by influencing one's location along the elaboration likelihood continuum. That is, variables can influence persuasion by influencing the likelihood that recipients will either thoughtfully or non-thoughtfully process messages.

Motivational factors

As stated earlier, motivation to elaborate plays a crucial role in determining individuals are influenced. Variables that influence motivation can come from both individual differences and/or situation influences.

Individual differences
Perhaps one of the most studied individual differences in persuasion is the need for cognition (Cacioppo and Petty 1982; Cacioppo et al. 1984a, 1996). Need for cognition measures an individual's intrinsic enjoyment of and motivation to thoughtfully consider information. As such, individuals high in need for cognition enjoy elaborating, and demonstrate a proclivity to elaborate persuasive information, even when situational influences do not prompt such consideration. In contrast, individuals low in need for cognition do not enjoy elaborating, and tend to rely upon non-thoughtful persuasion processes (for example Cacioppo et al. 1986a).

Note, however, that individual differences in need for cognition do not necessarily entail differences in elaboration. Individuals low in need for cognition do elaborate when situational influences warrant such thoughtful consideration, and individuals high in need for cognition do not elaborate when situational factors reduce their ability to elaborate (see Cacioppo et al. 1996). Rather, individual differences in need for cognition establish a base line of elaboration likelihood, which can be influenced by situational factors. All else being equal, high need for cognition individuals are more likely to engage in thoughtful elaboration of persuasive messages than low need. Situational variables must also be considered, however, in predicting elaboration likelihood.[3]

Situational influences
Personal relevance (that is, *involvement*) has been found to be a fundamental situational variable that influences elaboration (Petty and Cacioppo 1979; Petty et al. 1983a; Petty and Cacioppo 1984, 1990; Johnson and Eagly 1989; Petty et al. 1992). To the extent that the persuasive message is presented in such a way as to increase perceptions of involvement, elaboration is likely to increase. For example, when message recipients are instructed that they will have the opportunity to select an advertised product (Petty et al. 1983a) or that a produced policy change (such as the requirement of passing a comprehensive exam to graduate from college: Petty et al. 1981a) will directly influence message recipients, they are more likely to elaborate than if they are instructed that they will not have an opportunity to select the advertised product or that the produced policy changes will not influence them. Research

has suggested that involvement can be manipulated in many, often subtle ways. For example, Burnkrant and Unnava (1989) found that by changing advertisements such that they referred to 'you' (that is, second person singular tense) rather than 'one' or 'people' involvement and elaboration increased.

Since the advent of the ELM, many situational factors have been found that influence motivation to elaborate. Whether people believe that they alone are or instead are part of a group that is responsible for evaluating a message influences motivation to elaborate (Petty et al. 1980). Similarly, whether people believe that a position is advocated by one or multiple sources influences motivation to elaborate (Harkins and Petty 1981, 1987). Other variables found to influence motivation to elaborate include surprise (Maheswaran and Chaiken 1991; Baker and Petty 1994; Petty et al. 2001), messages authored by stigmatized sources (Petty et al. 1999), expectation of future social interaction (Chaiken 1980), loss of control (Pittman 1993), feelings of ambivalence about the message topic (Maio et al. 1996) and perceived scarcity of the attitude object (Bozzolo and Brock 1992).

Ability factors

A number of variables influence ability to elaborate. *Distraction* is one. When individuals are distracted, they are less able to expend the cognitive effort necessary to elaborate persuasive messages. As a result, they are more likely to rely upon non-thoughtful processes (see Petty et al. 1976; Petty and Brock 1981). The extent to which the information in the persuasive message is available has also been found to influence ability to elaborate. The greater the information availability, as a function of such variables as message repetition (Cacioppo and Petty 1989) and rate of speech of the communicator (Smith and Shaffer 1995), the greater the ability of message recipients to thoughtfully consider issue-relevant information. Other variables found to influence ability include recipient posture (Petty et al. 1983b), time pressure (Ratneshwar and Chaiken 1991), and physiological arousal (Sanbonmatsu and Kardes 1988).

Multiple roles by which variables can influence persuasion

One of the unique and most powerful features of the ELM is the proposition that a variable can influence persuasion through different roles (see Postulate 3). Specifically, the ELM hypothesizes that when the overall elaboration likelihood is low, a variable can influence persuasion by relatively non-thoughtful processes. When the overall elaboration likelihood is moderate, a variable can influence persuasion by influencing the extent of elaboration. When the overall elaboration likelihood is high, a variable can influence persuasion by either influencing the direction of issue-relevant thoughts (that is, the variable biases the direction of elaboration) or a variable can influence persuasion by serving as an argument (see Petty and Cacioppo 1986; Petty et al. 1994; Petty and Wegener 1998, 1999).

To illustrate, recall that balance process theories of persuasion postulated that interpersonal attitudinal discrepancy can influence persuasion. The multiple role hypothesis suggests that this variable could influence persuasion through different roles, depending upon the elaboration likelihood. Under conditions of low elaboration likelihood, interpersonal attitudinal discrepancy is predicted by the ELM to most likely change attitudes through a relatively non-thoughtful process. For example, you might simply decide to agree with a friend, without thoughtfully considering the issue-relevant merits of the attitude (for example Cacioppo and Petty 1981). Alternatively, under conditions of moderate elaboration likelihood, interpersonal attitudinal discrepancy might prompt thoughtful consideration. For example, you might discover that a friend holds an attitude different from yours, and this discrepancy might lead you to consider thoughtfully the basis of your attitude.

Under conditions of high elaboration likelihood, interpersonal attitudinal discrepancy could either influence the nature of your thoughts, or instead serve as an argument. For example, you might be motivated to hold an attitude that is similar to your friend, and as a consequence, elaborate attitude-relevant information in a manner that produces such agreement. That is, the cognitive responses that you generate are likely to be biased to agree with your friend, and attitude change is based upon these biased thoughts. Alternatively, if your friend's attitude can be construed as being related to the merits of the attitude, you might use your friend's attitude as an argument in your thoughtful consideration of your evaluation. The ELM advances the notion, then, that the same variable is hypothesized to be able to influence persuasion through different variables, depending upon the elaboration likelihood (see Petty et al. 1994; Petty and Wegener 1998; Fleming and Petty 1999; Petty and Wegener 1999).

Trustworthiness

Priester and Petty (forthcoming) provide evidence that perceptions of source trustworthiness (coupled with high expertise) can influence persuasion by different roles. Priester and Petty reasoned that if a message recipient can be confident that an expert source will be willing to provide accurate information because of his or her high trustworthiness, they may forgo the effortful task of scrutinizing the message and, instead, unthinkingly accept the conclusion as valid. In contrast, if a message recipient is unsure as to whether an expert source will provide accurate information because of the sources low or questionable trustworthiness, they may feel the need to scrutinize the arguments to ascertain if the communication is indeed cogent and valid. Thus, trustworthiness influences a person's assurance of accuracy. And this assurance of accuracy is hypothesized to lead to differences in thoughtful elaboration of the persuasive message.

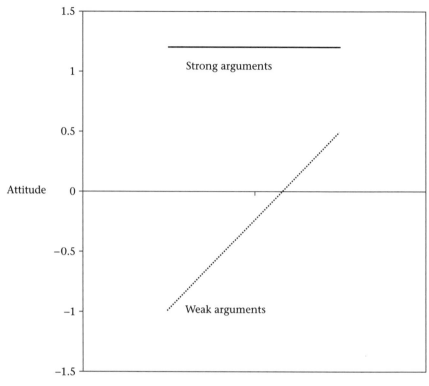

Figure 5.2   Attitude as a function of endorser trustworthiness and argument quality (Priester and Petty, forthcoming, Experiment One)

In this research, source trustworthiness was manipulated by both using familiar endorsers who differed in terms of trustworthiness (Experiment One) and by manipulating background information on unfamiliar endorsers to create different perceptions of trustworthiness (Experiment Two). To make inferences of the persuasion processes, both the manipulation of argument quality and the assessment of cognitive responses were employed. The attitude results of Experiment One are graphed in Figure 5.2.

The results provide evidence for two distinct processes by which source trustworthiness can influence attitudes. First, source trustworthiness influenced the extent of elaboration. When source trustworthiness was low, recipients engaged in greater product related elaboration than when source trustworthiness was high. Under low source trustworthiness, argument quality had a larger impact on attitudes and product focused thoughts were more highly correlated with attitudes than when source trustworthiness was high.

Second, source trustworthiness served as a simple cue when perceptions of high trustworthiness reduced message elaboration. That is, when the endorser was perceived as trustworthy, not only did this attenuate the impact of argument quality and message-based thinking, but attitudes tended to be influenced by *how trustworthy* recipients perceived the source to be. Specifically, a profile of the product-related cognitive responses revealed that these thoughts predicted the attitudes associated with the untrustworthy endorser ($r = 0.60$) more than the attitudes associated with the trustworthy endorser ($r = 0.25$). In contrast, the attitudes associated with the trustworthy endorser were more highly correlated with a measure assessing how trustworthy the endorser was perceived to be ($r = 0.43$) than the attitudes associated with the untrustworthy endorser ($r = 0.11$).

Examine Figure 5.2. You will note that the attitudes associated with strong arguments do not differ in terms of extremity. One possible conclusion, if one were to use only strong arguments, is that trustworthiness does not influence persuasion. However, consideration of the processes underlying these two, apparently similar attitudes, reveals that trustworthiness influenced the process by which these attitudes were formed. The attitude resulting from an advertisement endorsed by an untrustworthy source were based more upon thoughtful elaboration of the issue-relevant merits of the product, whereas the attitude resulting from an advertisement endorsed by a trustworthy source were based more upon non-thoughtful acceptance of the message. As we will explain below, such differences are important for both theoretical and applied reasons.

Mood

An individual's mood has also been found to influence persuasion by **multiple roles** (see Petty et al. 1994; Petty and Wegener 1998, 1999). Petty et al. (1993a) examined how mood influences persuasion under conditions of high and low elaboration likelihood. Petty et al. (1993a) conducted two studies, in which they used convergent methods to vary positive and neutral mood, and motivation to think. In both studies, positive mood led to greater persuasion than neutral mood, regardless of motivation to think. However, the process by which mood influenced attitudes differed as a function of the manipulations to think.

As predicted by the ELM, when individuals were not motivated to think, attitude change was the direct result of participants' mood. Specifically, mood influenced attitudes without influencing cognitive responses. In contrast, when individuals were motivated to think, mood influenced the generation of thoughts in response to the message, and these cognitive responses influenced attitude. Not surprisingly, mood did not influence attitudes directly when individuals were motivated to thoughtfully process the persuasive information. Thus, mood influenced persuasion by different roles, depending upon whether the elaboration likelihood was high or low.

But what about conditions of moderate elaboration likelihood? Can mood also influence the extent of elaboration? Wegener et al. (1995) examined this question and found that positive mood can both foster and hinder the extent of thoughtful consideration, depending upon whether the persuasive information appears to be pleasant or unpleasant. Specifically, when the message topic is expected to be unpleasant, individuals in a happy mood reduce the amount of thoughtful elaboration, whereas when the message topic is expected to be pleasant, individuals in a happy mood increase the amount of thoughtful elaboration. This pattern of influences can be readily understood by proposing that individuals wish to maintain a positive mood. As such, elaborating happy information and avoiding unhappy information provides one mechanism by which to regulate mood (Wegener and Petty 1994). Thus, mood can influence persuasion by multiple roles, depending upon the overall elaboration likelihood.

The influences of variables on persuasion

When the implications of multiple roles are fully understood, it becomes apparent that conceptualizing variables (such as source features) as either peripheral cues or message arguments is misguided (see Petty et al. 1987, 1993b). Rather, the power of the ELM is that it provides the insight that the same variable can influence persuasion by different roles, depending upon the overall elaboration likelihood. Thus, although a source characteristic is likely to serve as a peripheral cue under conditions of low elaboration likelihood, that same source characteristic is likely to serve as an argument (if relevant to the issue) or bias thoughts under conditions of high elaboration likelihood. That same source characteristic may accentuate or attenuate elaboration under conditions of moderate elaboration likelihood.

Resolution of conflicting research findings

Recall that one tension underlying persuasion research was the apparent conflicting nature of many of the findings. Findings that variables can sometimes increase persuasion, sometimes decrease persuasion, and sometimes appear not to influence attitudes at all mystified researchers. The ELM provides a theory by which to understand how this situation arises, and by which to predict when variables will lead to increases or decreases in persuasion. For example, when a variable influences the extent of elaboration, the nature of the arguments will determine whether that variable is associated with increased or decreased persuasion.

Consider the case of distraction. If distraction is examined using arguments that would normally generate positive cognitive responses, then distraction will be found to reduce persuasion. That is, more distraction results in less persuasion. This reduction in persuasion is due to the fact that distraction reduces the ability of the person to generate and be persuaded by positive cognitive responses. But what if distraction is examined using arguments that would normally generate negative cognitive responses? In this circumstance, distraction will be found to increase persuasion. That is, more distraction results in greater persuasion. Of course, this increase in persuasion is due to the fact that distraction reduces the ability of the person to generate and be persuaded by negative cognitive responses. Thus, distraction can either increase or decrease persuasion.

Consider the case of trustworthiness. That variables can influence persuasion by different roles sheds light on the conflicting findings reported by Hovland et al. (1953). Specifically, a trustworthy source should be expected to lead to greater persuasion, when the message is composed of weak arguments. And a trustworthy source might lead to less or equivalent attitude change when the message is composed of strong arguments. Importantly, the ELM allows one to understand when and why trustworthiness is likely to influence persuasion. Thus, the ELM provides a theory that unifies and clarifies prior conflicting research results.

Consequences of elaboration

Thus far, we have outlined how the ELM posits that attitudes can be formed and/or changed by one of two, qualitatively different psychological processes. Attitudes can be changed as a result of relatively effortful consideration of the merits central to the persuasive message, in which case the subsequent attitudes are the result of cognitive responses to the information. Attitudes can alternatively be changed as a result of relatively non-thoughtful processes, in which case the subsequent attitudes are the result of pairing the attitude with a cue, that is not diagnostic of the central merits of the persuasive information.

We have also presented the two methods most commonly used in order to assess differences in elaboration. Differences in elaboration can be inferred by examining the cognitive responses to the persuasive information. Differences in either the amount, nature, or relationship of the thoughts to the attitudes are indicative of differences in elaboration at the time of attitude formation or change. Differences in elaboration can alternatively be inferred by manipulating the quality of the arguments to which research participants are exposed. Greater differences between attitudes resulting from exposure to the strong and weak arguments (that is, greater argument quality differentiation) suggests that the attitudes were formed or changed under conditions of greater elaboration.

We have just presented an outline of the different roles by which variables can influence persuasion. Under conditions of low elaboration likelihood, variables can influence persuasion by serving as peripheral cues. Under conditions of moderate elaboration likelihood, variables can influence persuasion by influencing either the motivation and/or ability of individuals to elaborate the persuasive information. Under conditions of high elaboration likelihood, variables can influence persuasion by either serving as arguments, or by influencing the valence of the cognitive responses. This shows how the ELM resolves prior conflicting research findings.

Theoretical importance of elaboration

All of this theoretical framework is based upon the proposition that the key difference in how attitudes are changed is whether the process is one of thoughtful elaboration of issue-relevant information or instead whether the process is one of relatively less thoughtful processes based. A concern not addressed, up to this point, is why elaboration plays such a crucial theoretical role. After all, there exist many possible differences in the processes that are all categorized as non-thoughtful. Why not advance additional distinctions between persuasion processes, such as whether the process is non-thoughtful because of associative processes (such as classical conditioning) or instead non-thoughtful because of inferences (such as heuristics)? That is, one could argue that persuasion researchers should conceptualize more than two-routes. Similarly, at a general level, all persuasion, regardless of process, engages some form of cognitive activity. As such, why not conceptualize that all persuasion is the result of one route (Kruglanski and Thompson 1999; Kruglanski et al. 1999; see also Kunda 1999; Smith and DeCoster 1999).

The answer to why the ELM differentiates processes according to whether the process is based upon thoughtful elaboration or non-thoughtful processes rests upon the attitudinal consequences of the processes. In this section, we will explain how **thoughtful attitude change** processes result in attitudes that differ in meaningful and important ways from attitudes that are the result of relatively non-thoughtful persuasion processes. Basically, attitudes that are formed or changed as a result of relatively thoughtful elaboration are more likely to come to mind faster, persist over a longer period of time, resist counterpersuasive efforts, and to guide behaviour than attitudes that are formed or changed as a result of relatively non-thoughtful processes.

In short, attitudes that are the result of thoughtful elaboration possess greater **attitude strength** than attitudes that are not the result of elaboration (see Petty and Krosnick 1995; Petty et al. 1995b). In this chapter we will explain why these differences are hypothesized to occur and provide evidence supporting each of the differences.

Attitude structure

Consider the process of elaboration. When people elaborate persuasive information, they consider the central merits of an argument, often compare that information not only to their prior attitude, but also compare and integrate that information with prior knowledge that they have on the topic, and perhaps even compare and integrate that information with other, related topics. As such, elaboration is hypothesized to change an individual's cognitive structure, such that there are more associations and linkages with an elaborated than unelaborated attitude object (Petty and Cacioppo 1986; see also Srull 1981; Srull et al. 1985; Hamilton et al. 1989). It is these structural dimensions that are hypothesized to underlie the differences that result from thoughtful versus **non-thoughtful attitude change** processes. Although attitude structure and function received a great deal of attention in the 1980s (for example Pratkanis et al. 1989), the question of how to measure and assess structural issues related to attitude strength is still relatively unexplored.

Accessibility

Imagine if you will, that at breakfast one morning, your room-mate asks if you would like to eat a specific breakfast cereal. How quickly your attitude comes to mind, when presented with the attitude object (in this case, the question), has been found to be an important dimension of attitudes. For some people, their attitude towards that breakfast cereal might come to mind quickly. For others, their attitude towards that breakfast cereal might come to mind slowly, if at all. Research has demonstrated that those individuals for whom the attitudes come to mind faster are better able to use their attitudes in a variety of ways. For example, when attitudes come to mind faster, people are able to make decisions quicker, and those decisions are less stressful (Fazio et al. 1992a; Blascovitch et al. 1993). In addition, research has provided support for the notion that individuals with chronically faster attitudes are able to adapt to stressful new environments better than individuals with chronically slower attitudes (Fazio and Powell 1997).

The speed with which an attitude comes to mind upon the presentation of an attitude object is called attitude accessibility. Fazio (1995) has conducted a programme of research examining both the antecedents and consequences of accessibility. Highly accessible attitudes are more likely to guide thinking (Fazio and Williams 1986; Houston and Fazio 1989), more likely to guide behaviour (Fazio and Williams 1986), and even more likely to guide perception (Roskos-Ewoldsen and Fazio 1992) than attitudes that are not as accessible (see Fazio (1995) for a review).

Given that attitudes that are formed as the result of elaboration are hypothesized to have more associations and to have more linkages than attitudes that are formed as the result of non-thoughtful processes, it seems reasonable that elaborated attitudes should be more accessible than non-elaborated attitudes (Petty and Cacioppo 1986).

Recent research has supported this notion. Priester and Petty (2002, study 2) manipulated the perceived trustworthiness of an unfamiliar source. As discussed earlier, sources who are perceived to possess expertise but also be of questionable trustworthiness are more likely to prompt elaboration than sources who are perceived to possess expertise and are also perceived to be of high trustworthiness. In fact, the Trustworthiness X Argument Quality interaction and the correlations between cognitive responses and attitudes supported the notion that individuals elaborated the advertisement endorsed by the untrustworthy celebrity more than the advertisement endorsed by the trustworthy celebrity. Of greater importance for the present discussion, however, is that the accessibility of the attitudes toward the product featured in the advertisement was also assessed. As predicted by the ELM, individuals who were presented with the advertisement endorsed by the untrustworthy endorser were able to report their attitudes faster than the individuals who were presented with the advertisement endorsed by the trustworthy endorser. That is, trustworthiness influenced the extent to which participants elaborated the advertisement, and the extent of elaboration influenced the extent to which the attitudes were accessible (see also Petty et al. 1995a, 1995b).

Persistence

Imagine that while relaxing at home one evening you watch a television commercial advertising a breakfast cereal. Advertisers hope that your attitude will be changed to be more favourable toward the cereal as a consequence of having watched the commercial. But for how long will your attitude remain changed? Long enough to last until your next shopping trip?

As was discussed earlier, the question of attitude persistence has been of interest to persuasion researchers since the 1930s. Recall that Peterson and Thurstone (1933, 1970) exposed junior high and high school students to different films. For four out of five of the films, they found that attitudes were most influenced by the film immediately after exposure to the film, and that as time passed, the influence of the film on the attitudes diminished. This is the classic finding in attitude literature: Attitude change decays over time. Researchers have observed this effect repeatedly, and some have even despaired at the limited effects of persuasion over time (Cook and Flay 1978).

The ELM hypothesizes that, although attitudes are likely to decay over time, the relative rate of decay is influenced by the process by which the attitude is formed or changed. Attitudes that are formed or changed as the result of thoughtful elaboration are hypothesized to decay more slowly (stated differently, to persist longer) than attitudes that are formed or changed as the result of non-thoughtful processes. The literature on attitude persistence reveals that a number of variables have been found to moderate the rate of attitude decay. For example, Elms (1966) found that self-generated arguments lead to greater persistence. Johnson and Watkins (1971) found that increased message repetitions lead to greater persistence. Watts and Holt (1979) found that absence of distraction leads to greater persistence. Ronis et al. (1977) found that the use of involving topics leads to greater persistence. Haugtvedt and Petty (1992) found that individuals high in need for cognition showed greater persistence than individuals low in need for cognition. Each of these manipulations can be conceptualized as providing greater motivation and/or opportunity to elaborate the persuasive information. Thus, each of the studies can be seen as providing evidence that supports the notion that attitudes changed as the result of elaboration are more likely to persist longer over time than attitudes changed as the result of non-thoughtful processes. As such, your attitude toward the cereal is likely to persist longer if you elaborate the information from the commercial than if you accept the information in a non-thoughtful manner.

But what of the surprising result found by Peterson and Thurstone (1933, 1970)? Recall that for one of the movies, the influence of the film was greater after a period of time than immediately after viewing the film. In fact, this seemingly anomalous result has been found by other researchers, and given the name 'the sleeper effect'. The sleeper effect is said to occur when immediately after persuasion attitudes are not as influenced as they are later in time. That is, attitudes become more, rather than less, favourable toward the persuasive message over time. The ELM provides an explanation for when and why the sleeper effect occurs. According to the ELM, the sleeper effect is most likely to occur when a persuasive message has been elaborated, but following this elaboration there is a discounting cue suggesting that the persuasive message is somehow flawed or inaccurate. As such, the resulting attitude has the structural properties associated with strong attitudes, but the discounting cue temporarily attenuates the changed attitude. Over time, the effect of the discounting cues dissipates, and the persistence of the underlying changed attitude emerges (see Priester et al. 1999).

Resistance

Return again, to your relaxing evening watching television during which you are presented with a commercial for a breakfast cereal. As a result of watching this commercial, your attitude changes. You now evaluate the cereal favourably. We have just examined the question of how long your attitude will persist. We have not examined the question, however, of the influence of other commercials. Specifically if you sit in front of the television long enough, there undoubtedly will come another commercial advertising a different breakfast cereal. How likely is your attitude toward the initial cereal likely to change as a result of being exposed to this commercial for a competing brand? That is, how resistant is your attitude to subsequent attempts to change it?[4]

The question of **attitude resistance** has received considerable research (for example Lewan and Stotland 1961; McGuire and Papageorgis 1961; McGuire 1964; Pfau et al. 1990; Bassili 1996). The ELM predicts that attitudes that are changed or formed as the result of thoughtful elaboration are more likely to resist counterpersuasive attempts than attitudes that are the result of non-thoughtful persuasion processes. Haugtvedt and Petty (1992) found that individuals high in need for cognition were more likely to resist subsequent attacks to the attitude than individuals low in need for cognition. Haugtvedt and Wegener (1994) found that individuals who were exposed to a message of high personal relevance (and consequently more likely to elaborate the information) were more likely to be persuaded by an initial message and to rebuff a second, contradicting message than those individuals who were exposed to a message of low personal relevance (and consequently less likely to elaborate the information). In both Haugtvedt and Petty (1992) and Haugtvedt and Wegener (1994), evidence suggests that the individuals who possessed attitudes that were the result of elaboration were more likely to counter-argue the information in the second, attacking message than the individuals who possessed attitudes that were the result of non-thoughtful attitude change processes.

It appears, then, that the structural properties associated with attitudes that are the result of elaboration allow individuals to use their knowledge and beliefs to counter-argue the information contained in counterpersuasive attempts. Thus, your attitude toward the breakfast cereal is most likely to resist the counterpersuasive advertising of competing cereals if you elaborate the information contained in the advertisement for the initial breakfast cereal.

Behavioural intention and behaviour

Recall that at the outset of this chapter, we explained that part of the importance placed on the concept of attitudes can be attributed to the influence that attitudes are presumed to have on behaviour. Attitudes are often conceptualized as mediating behaviour. To illustrate, return one last time to your evening of leisure, watching the television and encountering the commercial for the breakfast cereal. The hope of the advertisers for the cereal is that as a result of changing your attitude to be positive toward the cereal, you will at some point purchase the cereal. But will you?

The question of if and when attitudes guide behaviour is a long and knotted trail. There is a tradition of researchers finding evidence that (sometimes) attitudes do not predict behaviour (for example LaPierre 1934; Bray 1950; Kutner, Wilkins, and Yarrow 1952; DeFleur and Westie 1958; Festinger 1964; Linn 1965; Berg 1966; Warner and DeFleur 1969; Wicker 1969). This research culminated in a crisis in the late 1960s, at which time one researcher suggested that the attitude construct be abandoned entirely due to its inability to predict behaviour (Wicker 1969).

The ELM predicts that attitudes that are changed as the result of elaboration are more likely to guide behavioural intentions and behaviour than attitudes that are changed as the result of non-thoughtful processes. Petty et al. (1983) explored the relation among motivation to elaborate, presence of a persuasive cue, the resulting attitude change processes and the properties associated with the resulting attitudes. With this experiment, it is possible to explore the influence of elaboration on behavioural intention. Motivation to elaborate was manipulated by exposing participants to an advertisement that either suggested that the product would be available (high elaboration) or not available (low elaboration) in the participant's town. In addition, participants were informed that they could choose a gift, either which included (high elaboration) or did not include (low elaboration) the advertised product. In order to assess differences in elaboration, the quality of the arguments provided for the product were manipulated to be strong or weak.

This study found that attitudes formed as a result of thoughtful elaboration were associated with greater attitude-behavioural intention correspondence than attitudes formed as a result of non-thoughtful persuasion processes. Specifically, attitudes changed by thoughtful consideration of the persuasive information contained in the advertisement exhibited a higher correlation between attitudes and purchase intention ($r = 0.59$) than did attitudes changed by less thoughtful processes ($r = 0.36$). Thus, this experiment provides evidence consistent with the notion that attitudes that are formed or changed as the result of elaboration are more likely to guide behavioural intentions than attitudes that are formed as the result of non-thoughtful persuasion processes.

Although the results of the Petty et al. (1983) study demonstrates that whether a persuasive message has been elaborated or instead non-thoughtfully processed moderates the influence of attitudes on behavioural intention, it does not demonstrate that this difference in persuasion processes moderate the influence of attitudes on behaviour itself. Fortunately, Cacioppo et al. (1986) provide such a demonstration. They (1986) investigated whether the attitudes of those individuals who were high in need for cognition influenced behaviour to a greater extent than those individuals who were low in need for cognition. Recall that need for cognition is an individual difference associated with chronic differences in likelihood to elaborate. Individuals high in need for cognition enjoy thinking, and thus are more likely to thoughtfully consider issue-relevant information, whereas individuals low in need for cognition do not intrinsically enjoy thinking, and thus are likely to engage in thoughtful consideration of issue-relevant information only when prompted to by situational influences, such as personal relevance, surprise (Petty et al. forthcoming), and untrustworthy endorsers (Priester and Petty 1995; see Cacioppo et al. 1996).

Cacioppo et al. (1983) surveyed college students approximately 8 weeks prior to the 1984 presidential election. At this time, students were asked to provide their attitudes towards the candidates in addition to completing the need for cognition scale (Cacioppo et al. 1984). On the three evenings following the election, the students were contacted by phone and were asked for whom they voted. As predicted by the ELM, the attitudes of the students who were high in need for cognition were more influential in guiding voting behaviour than the attitudes of the students who were low in need for cognition. Specifically, the correlation between the attitudes for the students high in need for cognition and their voting behaviour was $r = 0.87$, whereas the correlation between the attitudes for the students low in needs for cognition and their voting behaviour was $r = 0.46$.

Although the Cacioppo et al. (1983) findings provide support for the prediction provided by the ELM, they rely on an indicator of elaboration that is based upon an individual difference, rather than a manipulation. As such, one can always argue that difference other than elaboration, between the high and low need for cognition students, could explain the results (although it should be pointed out that other possible factors were examined and controlled for in the study). More conclusive evidence would be provided by a study in which elaboration likelihood is manipulated, and this manipulation results in differential influence of attitudes on behaviour.

Priester et al. (2001) provide such a study; they investigated the influence of elaboration on choice. In their study, all participants were exposed to an advertisement for a fictitious candy bar. This advertisement contained both strong arguments and positive features that could serve as peripheral cues. As a consequence of this combination of potential arguments and peripheral cues, it was predicted that individuals would form a positive attitude toward the candy bar regardless of the process by which the attitude was formed. Those participants who were thoughtfully paying attention to the arguments would form a positive attitude as a result of the positive cognitive responses that resulted from the strong arguments. Those participants who were forming attitudes by non-thoughtful processes would form a positive attitude as a result of the several peripheral cues (for example the advertisement contained many reasons to like the candy bar).

Half of the participants were asked to view the advertisement under conditions likely to foster thoughtful consideration of the issue-relevant information. Specifically, these participants were asked to pay attention to the thoughts and feelings that they experienced as they read the advertisement. The other participants were asked to view the advertisement under conditions likely to foster non-thoughtful attitude change processes. Specifically, these participants were asked to count the number of words that contained more than one syllable as they read the advertisement. It was thought, and pre-testing confirmed, that the former condition would lead to increased elaboration, whereas the latter condition (because of distraction) would lead to decreased elaboration (Figure 5.3).

After viewing the advertisement, participants provided their attitudes toward the candy bar. Attitudes did not differ as a function of elaboration manipulation: the attitudes of those who thoughtfully and of those who non-thoughtfully considered the advertisement were equally positive. Approximately ten minutes later, participants were provided with an opportunity to choose a candy bar. Although the attitudes were equally positive, the individuals who had elaborated the advertisement were more likely to choose the advertised candy bar than the individuals who had non-thoughtfully processed the advertisement. Thus, this experiment provides support for the proposition that elaboration moderates the influence of attitudes on behaviour. The attitudes that were formed as a result of thoughtful elaboration guided behaviour more than the attitudes that were formed as a result of non-thoughtful persuasion processes.

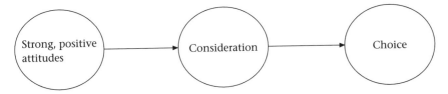

Figure 5.3 Mediational role of consideration on the attitude to behaviour relationship

In addition to measuring choice, Priester et al. (2001) also assessed whether participants considered the advertised product prior to choice. Recently, the concept of consideration has received a great deal of attention (for a review, see Roberts and Lattin 1997). In short, consideration has been found to play a role in many marketing-related phenomena (e.g. Kardes et al. 1993; Nowlis and Simonson 2000). Priester et al. (2001) sought to understand if elaboration influenced consideration, as well as choice. Their findings suggested that not only did elaboration influence consideration in addition to choice, but that consideration mediates the influence of elaboration on choice. Specifically, attitude objects associated with strongly held positive attitudes are more likely to be chosen than attitude objects associated with either weakly held positive attitude or negative attitudes (see Fazio et al. 1989). Mediational analyses performed on the Priester et al. (2001) data provide support for the idea that this influence is mediated, at least in part, by consideration. That is, attitude objects associated with strongly held positive attitudes are more likely to be considered, and it is this consideration that at least in part leads to choice. This relationship is presented in Figure 5.3.

Summary of research on consequences

The ELM provides a theoretical perspective that integrates the two questions of how attitudes are formed and changed with the question of when attitudes are likely to have consequences.[5] Whether an attitude is formed or changed by thoughtful elaboration of the issue-relevant information or is instead non-thoughtfully formed or changed influences attitude accessibility, persistence, resistance and ability to guide behaviour. These consequences provide the rationale for distinguishing between thoughtful elaboration and non-thoughtful attitude change processes. Although there are several different mechanisms hypothesized to underlie non-thoughtful persuasion processes, they all share the similarity of not only being the result of attitude change that does not focus on issue-relevant information, but also resulting in attitudes that are relatively weak. It should also be pointed out that the consequences that stem from differences in persuasion process also help resolve past (for example when attitudes guide behaviour) and present (for example how judgements are formed) empirical contradictions and theoretical tensions.

Conclusion

The field of persuasion is both historically and theoretically rich. Our understanding of how variables influence persuasion has become more sophisticated as new theories of persuasion have been advanced. The field has progressed from investigating main effect predictions of variables on persuasion (for example McGuire 1969, 1985) to conceptualizing variables as being able to influence persuasion through a number of processes (see Petty and Wegner 1998). This conceptual maturation has provided a coherent theoretical framework by which to understand apparently contradictory and baffling persuasion results. This conceptual maturation has also provided a framework for non-persuasion researchers. Specifically, there has emerged a bounty of dual-route models to explain different psychological phenomena (see Chaiken and Trope 1999). Thus, what started as a framework by which to resolve and better understand how attitudes are formed and changed has emerged as a dominant theory applicable to a wide variety of social behaviours.

Notes

1 Thurstone (1928), it should be noted, was the first to provide a method by which to measure attitudes.
2 Priester and Petty (2001) found that interpersonal attitudinal discrepancy (that is, agreement with one's enemies and disagreement with one's friends) can lead to increased feelings of evaluative tension (that is, ambivalence, see Priester and Petty 1996) in addition to or instead of attitude change.
3 Other individual differences have been found to influence elaboration likelihood. For example, Wood and colleagues (for example Wood et al. 1985; Kallgren and Wood 1986; Wood and Kallgren 1988) have examined how individual differences in issue-related knowledge influence elaboration. Their findings suggest that individuals with more knowledge are more likely to elaborate than individuals with less knowledge.
4 It should be noted that the ELM does not predict that all of the consequences are influenced. Rather the ELM predicts that the consequences can be independent (see Petty and Cacioppo 1986; Petty and Wegener 1998, 1999). For example, persistent attitudes are not necessarily resistant, and resistant attitudes are not necessarily persistent.
5 The ELM has also been used in order to address a controversy within the domain of judgements. Specifically, there has been a wave of research suggesting that judgements (and behaviour) are based upon construction processes (for example Tesser 1978; Bettman et al. 1998; Schwarz 1998, 1999). These researchers argue that individuals base their judgements upon information that is salient at the time of judgement. Subtle manipulations, such as varying the ease with which information is retrieved, lead to changes in judgement. Based upon such findings, some researchers have suggested that attitudes, defined as internally stored evaluations, do not influence judgements. Nayakankuppum and Priester (2001) used the ELM to derive the prediction that attitudes formed or changed as the result of elaboration should be more likely to influence judgements, and that attitudes formed or

changed as a result of non-thoughtful processes should be more likely to demonstrate the construction processes. A series of studies provided support for this prediction. Construction manipulations were more likely to influence attitudes formed under conditions of low elaboration likelihood, whereas stored evaluations were more likely to influence attitudes formed under conditions of high elaboration likelihood.

Suggested readings

Chaiken, S. and Trope, T. (eds) (1999) *Dual-Process Theories in Social Psychology*. New York: Guilford. Edited book in which contemporary social psychological theories that utilize a dual-process approach are presented.

Petty, R.E. and Cacioppo, J.T. (1981) *Attitudes and persuasion: Classic and Contemporary Approaches*. Dubuque, IA: William C. Brown. A text in which a history of persuasion is presented in order to develop and introduce the elaboration likelihood model of persuasion.

Petty, R.E. and Cacioppo, J.T. (1986) The elaboration-likelihood model of persuasion, in L. Berkowitz (ed.) *Advances in Experimental Social Psychology*, Vol. 19. New York: Academic Press. A highly cited chapter in which the elaboration likelihood model of persuasion is presented.

Petty, R.E. and Wegener, D.T. (1998) Attitude change: multiple roles for persuasion variables, in D. Gilbert, S. Fiske and G. Lindzey (eds) *Handbook of Social Psychology*, 4th edn. New York: McGraw-Hill. A chapter that elucidates the influence of variables on persuasion from the perspective of the elaboration likelihood model of persuasion.

6

Cognitive processes

We will review research on cognitive processes involved in consumer information processing. Specifically, we examine how consumers internally process
market-related information (for example product information, advertisements,
prices). First, we discuss how consumers attend to and form perceptions of
marketing stimuli. Then we examine how consumers categorize stimuli
in their environment and how they apply their category-based knowledge
(that is, schemas) when they form impressions. Next, we review literature on
memory processes and the effect of memory on judgements. Finally, we
discuss the processes by which consumers draw inferences and respond to
incomplete information.

Attention

Attention is the process by which an individual concentrates mental activity
on a stimulus. An important characteristic of attention is that it is selective.
That is, people attend to only certain stimuli and do not focus on others.
Social psychological research suggests that individuals attend to a stimulus
if the stimulus is personally relevant, unexpected, interesting and salient
(Kahneman 1973; McArthur and Post 1977; Nisbett and Ross 1980). For
example, people are more likely to pay attention to a person if that person
stands out by behaving in an unexpected way or by looking salient (for
example solo person of age group). Similarly, consumers were found to attend
to certain features in a product description when these features were made
salient in a usage situation (Ratneshwar et al. 1997). Moreover, unexpected
cues embedded in a message were found to prompt greater attention (Meyers-
Levy and Sternthal 1991). This effect was shown to vary as a function of
gender and the level of incongruity. Specifically, women as compared to men
had a lower threshold for elaborating on message cues. This difference was
eliminated when message cues prompted very little attention (for example

very low incongruity) or very high attention (for example very high incongruity). Subsequent research showed that processing goals influence the extent to which consumers pay attention to different types of cues (Shavitt et al. 1994). When consumers do not have specific processing goals, contextual factors such as scent or the material surrounding an object affects attention. For example, consumers spent more time looking at a focal object in an exploratory search task when the material surrounding that object was not very demanding (Janiszewski 1998). Morrin and Ratneshwar (2000) found that pleasant ambient scent increases consumers' attention to unfamiliar brand names, leading to improved recall.

There is also evidence that the first brand in a category attracts more attention than later entrants (Kardes and Kalyanaram 1992). In other words, consumers learn about the attributes of the first brand because these attributes will be perceived as novel and interesting. Since later entrants are likely to have similar attributes, information about the later entrants may be perceived as redundant and are less likely to attract attention. Consequently, consumers learn about the attributes of first more than they learn about the attributes of later entrants. Kardes and Kalyanaram (1992) found that order-of-entry effects were eliminated when subjects received information about the brands simultaneously as opposed to sequentially.

Consumers can attend to something in their peripheral vision even though they may not be aware of it (Janiszewski 1990). The non-conscious processing of stimuli in peripheral vision has been referred to as **preattentive processing** and can be explained on the basis of hemispheric resource theory (Allen 1983). When a stimulus is in peripheral vision, it is processed by the opposite hemisphere. For example, a stimulus presented in the right visual field is processed by the left hemisphere. Right hemisphere is suited for holistic, inferential processing (for example music, pictures, spatial information) and left hemisphere is suited for analytic, sequential, and repetitive processing (for example words, numbers) (Hansen 1981; Janiszewski 1988; Meyers-Levy 1989b). Consistent with hemispheric lateralization, Janiszewski (1988) found that subjects liked pictorial stimuli (for example pictorial ads) more when placed in the left, which encourages the use of holistic processing resources of the right hemisphere. Similarly, subjects liked verbal stimuli more when placed in the right, which encourages the use of analytic processing resources of the left hemisphere.

Preattentive processing can be improved due to the availability of increased resources in one hemisphere, which is a function of increased processing load in the other hemisphere (Friedman and Polson 1981; Janiszewski 1990). This has been referred to as the matching activation hypothesis and suggests that when individuals focus their attention on a certain task, preattentive processing associated with this task activates one hemisphere to a greater extent. The availability of resources in the other hemisphere also increases in anticipation of cooperative processing. Consistent with this hypothesis, Janizewski (1990) showed that an unfamiliar brand is preferred more when presented to the right of a picture. Processing pictures requires resources from the right hemisphere and in anticipation of cooperation, availability of resources in the other hemisphere (that is, left hemisphere) also increases. Increased resources in the left hemisphere improve preattentive processing of the brand name when the brand is placed in the right. Likewise, an unfamiliar brand is preferred more when presented to the left of verbal information. As preattentive processing increases, familiarity also increases and the fluency experienced during subsequent perception of the brand leads to more favourable evaluations of the brand. In another study, similar findings were obtained when pictorial or verbal information was placed in a peripheral visual field, suggesting that focal attention is not necessary for mere exposure-driven affective processes (Janizewski 1993).

Preattentive processing can also influence whether a brand will be included in the consideration set (Shapiro et al. 1997). Consumers were more likely to consider a brand for purchase as a result of preattentive processing although they did not have any memory of the brand. Further research suggested that inclusion of a brand in the consideration set as a function of incidental ad exposure can be explained based on perceptual and conceptual fluency effects (Shapiro 1999). Perceptual fluency suggests that exposure leads to a memory trace for the perceptual features of the stimulus (for example shape, brightness) and consequently, the features of the stimulus are more easily processed on a subsequent occasion. The ease of processing on a subsequent occasion leads to greater liking for the stimulus because perceivers misattribute ease of processing to familiarity and preference for the stimulus. Conceptual fluency suggests that incidental exposure may lead to increased liking or preference for semantically related stimulus, if incidental exposure involves the processing of semantic information.

In summary, previous research has examined both focal attention processes and preattentive processes. Consumers are more likely to attend to a stimulus, if the stimulus is unexpected, salient, and personally relevant. Processing goals and contextual factors also affect focal attention. Consumers can attend to something in their peripheral vision without being aware of it. Such preattentive processes were found to influence liking and consideration.

Perception

Perception is a process that uses previous knowledge to compile and interpret the stimuli that are registered by our senses (Matlin 1998). Previous academic research on consumer perception has focused on understanding how consumers perceive visual cues and prices and the effect of aural (for example music) and olfactory (for example scent) cues on consumer responses. Relatively little academic research investigated consumer perceptions through taste and touch (see Hornik 1992 for an exception).

Perception of visual cues

One of the most important factors in visual perception is colour. Recent research suggests that ads containing colours with higher levels of value (that is, lighter, pastel-like in appearance) and chroma (that is, rich and deep colour) lead to greater liking for the ad due to feelings of relaxation elicited by the higher value colour and feelings of excitement elicited by the higher chroma colour (Gorn et al. 1997). The effect of ad colour on persuasion was also found to depend on the correspondence between available and required processing resources (Meyers-Levy and Peracchio 1995). For example, when viewers devote few resources to processing, ads with some colour are more effective than black-and-white ads. In contrast, when resources devoted to ad processing are inadequate for thorough scrutiny, black-and-white ads and ads that highlight relevant aspects with colour were found more persuasive.

Another important factor in visual perception is volume. Research suggests that volume perceptions can influence consumption processes (Folkes et al. 1993; Raghubir and Krishna 1999). For example, Folkes et al. (1993) found that when the amount of supply could be assessed visually, consumers decreased their usage as supply decreased. However, this finding was limited to a certain range. Specifically, beyond an upper limit consumers did not increase their consumption and beyond a lower limit they did not decrease their consumption. In addition, they increased their consumption when supply was very limited. These findings were explained based on **assimilation** and contrast effects. A large supply increases product usage because consumers perceive a contrast between the supply and the amount poured. They increase their consumption so that the amount used does not seem small as compared to the supply. As the amount of supply decreases, the perceived contrast also decreases. At some point, consumers perceive the amount of supply and the amount adequate for a single use as similar, prompting subjects to use more due to assimilation effects.

Raghubir and Krishna (1999) examined the effect of package shape on perceived volume, perceived and actual consumption, post-consumption satisfaction and choice. In a series of experiments, they found that elongated containers were perceived to have higher volumes and these volume perceptions were invariant to processing ability and motivation manipulations. Specifically, subjects judged taller containers as having higher volumes even under high accuracy motivation and high ability conditions, suggesting that perceptual judgements may be partially automatic. However, when subjects started drinking from the containers, their experience contradicted their perceptions. In an effort to correct this discrepancy, subjects adjusted their perceived consumption and inferred that they consumed less from the elongated container. This lowered perceived consumption increased actual consumption. Their findings also indicated that subjects preferred an elongated container before consumption. However, post-consumption satisfaction was lower when the container was more (versus less) elongated.

In a retail setting, consumers rely on several visual cues to form judgements. When they enter a store or a shopping mall, judgements based on spatial perceptions are likely to be important in influencing choices. In forming spatial judgements, consumers were found to use the direct distance between the two points because of its high perceptual salience (Raghubir and Krishna 1996). Path direction and path angularity affect estimates of direct distance. When a path is unidirectional, the direct distance between its end points can be longer than a path that retraces its direction. Consequently, a path that retraces might be perceived as shorter than a path that is unidirectional although these two paths might be of the same length. Similarly, paths with wider angles are perceived to be longer than paths with narrow angles.

Consumers' store choices partly depend on perceptions of the assortment. Broniarczyk et al. (1998) examined factors that influence the perceptions of assortment and found that consumers may not notice a reduction in stock-keeping units (SKU) when they have lower preference for the items that were removed. Consumers were more likely to notice a reduction in SKUs, when their highly preferred items were removed. Broniarczyk et al. (1998) proposed that because size is an important cue in any perceptual representation, consumers are likely to notice any changes in the space allocated to the category. Consistent with this theorizing, they found that perceptions of assortment were lowered when the amount of space allocated to a category was reduced.

Perceptions of aural and olfactory cues

Aural cues
Research on the effects of aural cues on consumer behaviour has mostly focused on understanding the effect of background music in stores and in advertising. Interestingly, studies have shown that the tempo of the background music is positively related to the store traffic (Milliman 1986). Moreover, music with strong national associations led to increased sales of products from respective countries (North et al. 1999). Background music in advertisements may impair processing of brand information and comprehension particularly under incidental (versus goal-directed) learning tasks (Hoyer et al. 1984; Olsen 1997).

Olfactory cues
Pleasant ambient scents were found to increase liking for the store and the merchandise (Spangenberg et al. 1996). In addition, consumers perceive spending less time in a store with pleasant ambient scent as compared to a store with no scent. Pleasant ambient scents were also found to affect consumer decision making as a function of their congruity with the target product class (Mitchell et al. 1995). When the scent was congruent (versus incongruent)

with the product class, consumers were found to spend more time processing information and exhibit variety-seeking behaviour.

Price perceptions

According to adaptation level theory (Helson 1964), judgements depend on a comparison of the target with an adaptation level, which is a function of recent related experiences. For example, it has been proposed that consumers' price perceptions depend on a comparison of market prices with an internal reference price, which reflects an adaptation level of past prices (Greenleaf 1995; Kalyanaram and Winer 1995). In other words, attractiveness of a market price is determined by comparing it to an internal reference price. Janiszewski and Lichtenstein (1999) proposed that price perceptions may also depend on a comparison of market prices with an accessible price range. For example, $1.25 would be perceived as more favourable if accessible price range is $1.00–1.75 as compared to $0.75–1.50, keeping the average price constant across conditions. These predictions were generated on the basis of range theory (Volkmann 1951), which suggests a linear relationship between the stimulus range and the psychological scale individuals use to form their perceptions.

Consistent with range theory, Janiszewski and Lichtenstein (1999) found that the attractiveness of prices varied as a function of an accessible price range. Furthermore, endpoints of the price range were found to mediate the changes in attractiveness of prices. Since previous research has provided evidence consistent with both adaptation level theory and range theory, future research is necessary to investigate the factors that influence and psychological processes that underlie the use of an internal reference price versus an accessible price range.

In forming price perceptions, consumers utilize cues that would help them to judge the attractiveness of a price without extensive cognitive elaboration. For example, Alba et al. (1994) found that frequency cues affected price perceptions more than magnitude cues. In their experiments, subjects compared the prices of two stores, one with frequent but shallow discounts and one with infrequent but deep discounts. Although the average prices were equivalent, subjects perceived the prices at the store with frequent but shallow discounts more attractive. Subsequent research identified the conditions under which the depth versus the frequency of discounts influences price perceptions. Specifically, Alba et al. (1999) found that when processing price information was difficult (for example comparative prices exhibit complex and overlapping distributions), consumers utilized frequency of discounts in forming price perceptions. In contrast, when processing price information was easier (for example comparative prices have simple dichotomous distribution), a store with deeper discounts was perceived as having lower prices. The authors proposed that in the dichotomous condition, consumers may have anchored their sale-price judgement on the deep discount and then adjusted upward to estimate the regular price. Since the anchor was lower due to deep discounts, price perceptions were also lower compared to non-dichotomous condition. In the non-dichotomous condition, the depth of the discount was less vivid and frequency became the dominant cue. Future research can test these explanations directly to provide insight into the processes by which price perceptions are formed in complex environments with varying levels of promotional activity.

In summary, we have seen that perceptual processes affect consumer behaviour in a variety of settings. In particular, visual cues such as colour and volume, aural cues such as music, and olfactory cues such as ambient scent influence cognitive processes, attitudes and behaviour.

Categorization

Categorization refers to the process of assigning an instance to a particular group such as identifying a person as a salesperson or identifying a product as a Sony or a digital camera. Once a target is categorized, category knowledge is utilized in evaluations of that target (Sujan 1985). An object or a person can be categorized at different levels of abstraction. For example, a particular model of Ford Focus can be categorized as a car, as a sedan or as Ford. In addition to taxonomic categories, categories can be developed on the basis of consumers' goals (Barsalou 1985). Birthday gifts and vacation activities are examples of goal-derived categories. Depending on how products are categorized, different features may become important in consumers' evaluation. How do consumers categorize products, services, and other people? What are the determinants of category structure? In this section, we will review extant literature that addressed these questions.

Different views of category representation

The classical view, which was dominant until the 1970s, suggests that certain defining features or rules determine category membership. An instance should possess all of these defining features to be considered a member of the category. For example, to be categorized as a square, a shape must have four corners and four sides the same size. The classical view also implies that all category members are equally similar to each other. This view was disputed by later research, which pointed out that even simple categories (for example tables) can not be represented on the basis of such deterministic rules (Rosch 1978). Consequently, two general views (probabilistic and exemplar-based) were proposed to explain category representation. The probabilistic view suggests that categories are represented by a summary representation or an abstraction, referred to as a prototype (Rosch and Mervis 1975). Prototypes can be based on mean or modal values for relevant attributes or the single best example of the category. An instance is categorized based on its similarity to the prototype and similarity is assessed as an additive function over features. This view suggests that, like family members, category members share some features but there is no defining rule that applies to all members. This view also allows category members to vary in terms of their typicality. For example, car is a typical member of the vehicle category and scooter is less typical. Non-members also vary in their similarity to the category. Lawn mower is a better non-member of vehicle category than shovel. The fact that category members and non-members vary in their similarity to the category has been referred to as **graded structure** (Barsalou 1985).

One of the limitations of the standard prototype model is its assumption regarding the use of central tendency or abstraction in categorization. People also use other information such as correlation between features and variability of features across category members in classifying instances (Park and Hastie 1987). Exemplar-based models address these limitations and propose that categories are represented by sets of specific instances (Medin and Schaffer 1978). An instance is categorized to the extent that it activates multiple exemplars of that category and does not activate exemplars from alternative categories.[1] Because empirical research provided support for both views, several mixed-model representations have been proposed. For example, the exemplar-based abstraction view suggests that categorization may be based on exemplars but overtime people store an abstraction on the basis of these exemplars and may use that abstraction in categorization (Ross and Makin 1999).

Similarity plays an important role in understanding categories, but may not explain categorization adequately. A recent view suggests that category organization might be more likely to be guided by intuitive theories about how the world operates rather than similarity (Murphy and Medin 1985). Support for the theory based view comes from research in developmental psychology which suggests that category-based knowledge (that is, theories about category) overrides similarity-based judgements in children's categorization processes (Gelman and Markman 1986). In addition, research on goal-derived categories provide support for theory-based view by suggesting that people's knowledge about the world highlight similarities between instances that do not seem to be similar in the beginning (Barsalou 1985). It is possible that, particularly for broad brands (for example Sony, Toshiba), intuitive theories could play more important role in category organization than similarity of products.

Based on a review of alternative categorization models, Cohen and Basu (1987) proposed a contingency-based, mixed model approach to explain how consumers categorize products. According to Cohen and Basu (1987), consumers may use any of these representations (that is, rules, prototype or exemplar) initially to arrive at a quick judgement and can later make adjustments if necessary. Categorization processes can be automatic or deliberative and category representations can be employed based on analytical (that is, piecemeal processing of individual features) or non-analytical (that is, holistic) processes.[2] Their model suggests that consumers can use different representations of categories depending on contextual variables such as category learning context, task involvement/motivation, rule complexity and judgement setting. They propose that if category is learned through a definitional process, consumers are more likely to rely on rule-based and analytical processes in subsequent categorization. In contrast, if category is learned through exposure to exemplars, consumers are more likely to rely on exemplar-based and non-analytical processes in subsequent categorization. For example, doctors are probably more likely to use rule-based and analytical process in classifying different types of drugs, whereas patients are likely to rely on exemplar-based and non-analytical processes. There is also some evidence in social psychology, which suggests that initial learning about the category affects subsequent categorization. For example, Smith and Zarate (1990) found that subjects who learned about group prototypes before encountering individual group members were more likely to utilize prototype-based categorization processes, relative to subjects who learned about exemplars at the outset. Several interesting extensions can be envisioned in the context of consumption-related categories. For example, consumers may learn about a family brand through exposure to product advertisement (that is, exemplar-based) or through corporate advertisement that provides more abstract information. It is possible that consumers who are initially exposed to exemplars (versus abstract information) are likely to use different processes in evaluating brand extensions. Consumers who are initially exposed to exemplars may be more sensitive to product category similarity than those who are exposed to more abstract information.

Level of category

Studies have shown that categories can be represented at the basic (for example product type), subordinate (for example brand or specific products) and superordinate levels (for example product class: Sujan and Dekleva 1987). Whereas superordinate categories are generally described by abstract features, subordinate categories are associated with more specific features. Basic level categories have both abstract and specific features. People generally refer to the basic level categories such as 'chair' as opposed to 'furniture' (superordinate) or 'armchair' (subordinate) to identify objects. Also, discrimination within category members is minimized and between different categories is maximized at the basic level. Research showed that as the level of expertise increases, subordinate level becomes the basic level (Tanaka and Taylor 1991). Because of their knowledge, experts, compared to novices, can identify more attributes at the subordinate level and consequently can distinguish different instances with increased specificity (Alba and Hutchinson 1987).

Pendry and Macrae (1996) found that under high accountability (that is, when motivation is high), subjects are more likely to categorize people at a more differentiated subordinate level. This would imply that when consumers are highly involved they are more likely to use subordinate levels of categorization. For example, if a consumer is about to purchase a new car, instances are more likely to be categorized at the subordinate levels (for example Toyota Camry).

Measurement and determinants of typicality

Typicality has generally been operationalized using global measures that assess whether the instance is a good or a poor example, typical or atypical, representative or unrepresentative (Loken and Ward 1990). Typicality can also be measured at the attribute level (Viswanatan and Childers 1999). Respondents indicate the degree to which an instance is a good example of a particular category in terms of different attributes. Typicality is then calculated based on a combination of these attribute-based ratings. Typicality can also be measured indirectly at the attribute level. Specifically, respondents indicate the degree to which different attributes are characteristic of both an instance and a category. Across all attributes, the distance between the instance and the category can be used to calculate typicality ratings. Viswanatan and Childers (1999) showed that the attribute-level typicality measures perform better or as well as the global typicality measures.

Family resemblance is one determinant of typicality in categories and is defined as an exemplar's similarity to the central tendency of its category. The typicality of an exemplar increases as it shares more attributes with other members of the category. Family resemblance has generally been operationalized by asking research participants to list attributes of different members of a category. Family resemblance scores are calculated for a member based on the weighted sum of its attributes, where weights are determined by the number of category members who have the same attribute (Loken and Ward 1990).

Frequency of instantiation is another determinant of typicality. This refers to perceived estimates of how often an instance is encountered as a member of the category. It can be measured in two ways: frequency of encountering an instance across all contexts and frequency of encountering an instance in a specific context (Barsalou 1985). Barsalou defined 'familiarity' as frequency of instantiation across all contexts: 'familiarity is *category-independent* measure of frequency' and 'frequency of instantiation is category-specific measure of frequency' (Barsalou 1985: 681).

Barsalou (1985) also examined an exemplar's similarity to ideals associated with goals its category serves as a determinant of typicality. For example, in Barsalou's (1985) experiments, 'how happy people are to receive it' and 'how necessary it is to wear it' were ideal dimensions for birthday presents and clothing categories, respectively. Subjects rated each exemplar for its amount on its ideal dimension. Barsalou found that for taxonomic categories (for example animals, plants, furniture) family resemblance is an important determinant of typicality. However, for goal-derived categories, family resemblance did not predict typicality. Ideals and frequency of instantiation as a category member were significant determinants of typicality for both taxonomic and goal-derived categories. Familiarity was not significant in predicting typicality for both type of categories.

What are the determinants of typicality for product and brand categories? Does the level of a category influence the relationship between typicality and its determinants? Loken and Ward (1990) collected data for product and brand-level categories to address these questions and found that, across both subordinate and superordinate categories, typicality and family resemblance were correlated. In addition, common features significantly predicted both family resemblance and typicality. However, distinctive features were not related to family resemblance and did not significantly predict typicality for superordinate categories and were only weakly related with typicality for subordinate categories. Consistent with Barsalou's (1985) findings, frequency of instantiation, but not familiarity, determined typicality ratings. Attribute structure (that is, the degree to which the product has salient attributes related to the goals or uses of the category) and ideals were also found to be a significant determinant of typicality. Loken and Ward's (1990) findings also highlight how product/brand attitudes and typicality can be related. They found that attribute structure and attitudes better predicted typicality for subordinate than superordinate categories. Also, ideals and attribute structure moderated the relationship between attitude and typicality.

Do the determinants of typicality vary across different segments of consumers? A study by John and Sujan (1990) demonstrates that while younger children (4–5 years old) use perceptual cues (for example package related visual cues, size, colour, shape) in assessing typicality, older children (9–10 years old) use underlying attributes (for example taste, nutrition) in typicality judgements. Children at a certain developmental stage (for example 6–7 years old) use perceptual cues in categorization but are able to use underlying attributes as well when prompted. There is also some evidence that, unlike American children, Chinese children are less likely to rely on underlying attributes in grouping different sets of objects (Chiu 1972). Instead, Chinese children relied on relationships between objects in categorization. For example, they grouped mother and child together because the mother takes care of the baby.

There is also some evidence that males and females employ different processing styles in categorizing poor members of a category. Based on the premise that males' hemispheres are more lateralized, Meyers-Levy (1989a) found that priming of a visual (versus verbal) task activates males use of holistic processing style. When males used holistic processing style, they were more likely to judge poor members of the category as fitting well with the category. Because females' hemispheres were less lateralized, they were not very sensitive to manipulations that encourage the use of detailed or holistic processing.

Language is another important variable affecting typicality judgements (Schmitt and Zhang 1998). Classifiers are linguistic labels, which refer to shared properties of objects such as shape, size, thickness, elasticity and so on. Schmitt and Zhang (1998) collected data from native Mandarin and English speakers to examine how classifiers affect consumers' cognition and judgements. While classifiers are used in Mandarin, they are not used in English. Subjects provided similarity ratings for different sets of stimuli (for example gloves, shoes, scarf, belt). Results showed that Mandarin speakers, compared to English, rated object pairs sharing the same classifier more similar. In general, the results of these studies point out the importance of understanding cultural differences in consumer categorization.

Research suggests that affective processes have an impact on categorization. For example, Barone et al. (2000) demonstrated that positive mood enhances the perception of similarity between the core brand and the extension, leading to an improvement in the perceptions of the core brand company's competency to produce an extension, particularly for moderately incongruent extensions. These findings are consistent with previous research which suggests that positive mood promotes more flexible categorization (Isen and Daubman 1984; Kahn and Isen 1993).

Multiple categories

Instances can be associated with multiple groups. For example, in a consumer context, products often have multiple country-of-origin associations. A Japanese branded product can be made in Malaysia using parts made in Taiwan. How do people categorize objects when they can be associated with multiple categories?

Moreau et al. (2001b) investigated this issue in the context of really new products (for example digital camera, electric car). Such products can be interpreted using existing categories; however, multiple categories can be applied to infer their attributes. For example, for digital cameras, consumers use both the category of cameras and the category of scanners or computers. Moreau et al. (2001b) found that, when multiple categories are accessible, the first category activated tends to have a disproportionate impact on consumers' categorization and judgement. This is because once consumers transfer knowledge form the first category, consumers' ability to map information from a second category onto the really new product may be impaired. Their findings also suggest that this effect is reduced when relevant attribute information is clearly specified for each category. When consumers' knowledge transfer is guided by focused processing, they are likely to have higher ability to transfer relevant knowledge from the second category.

Research in person categorization indicates that accessible attitudes and diagnosticity of categories are important in understanding which category will be used when multiple categories are activated. For example, Smith et al. (1996) showed that if people have highly accessible attitudes toward a category, that particular category will be used to categorize instances associated with multiple categories. In contrast, Stangor et al. (1992) suggests that perceivers attend to most informative features of the target. They utilize the most diagnostic category-based information available for judgement. Perceivers also utilize combined memberships by the use of subgroups. Both accessibility and diagnosticity play an important role in categorizing instances with multiple categories.

Category-based induction

Do consumers use category knowledge and typicality assessments to induce attributes of category members? For example, if consumers learn that 'Sharp has reliable TVs', to what extent do they infer that other Sharp products are reliable? Research on **category-based induction** (for example Osherson et al. 1990) suggests that consumers are likely to generalize from one specific category (for example TVs) to a general category (for example all products) more readily than they generalize to another specific category (for example vacuum cleaners), which has been referred to as the inclusion effect. Joiner and Loken (1998) showed that consumers are viable to inclusion effects, but the effect is attenuated when the conclusion category is moderately typical.

In this section, we have reviewed different views of category representation, **category levels**, determinants of typicality and category-based induction. Next we discuss when and how consumers utilize their category knowledge in evaluating products and how such knowledge may be modified in response to incongruent information.

Schemas

Schemas are cognitive structures that represent organized knowledge about different categories such as self, other people, events and objects. Consumers have schemas about product categories, brands, country-of-origin, themselves as consumers, other consumers, marketing and sales tactics and so on (Folkes and Kiesler 1991). For example, a consumer's schema about Amazon.com may include product categories that are sold at Amazon, attributes such as wide assortment, fast service, reliability, recommendations, and overall evaluations. Similarly, a fruit juice schema may include attributes such as nutritious, all-natural, slightly sweet, made of fruit, and served cold (Meyers-Levy and Tybout 1989). The cognitive organization of information in a schema may depend on processing objectives. Park and Wyer (1994) found that subjects with an attribute judgement objective organized the information in memory in terms of attribute-item clusters. In contrast, subjects with an overall evaluation objective organized the information in memory in terms of both attribute-item clusters and a general evaluative concept of the product.

Consumers use schemas to classify products into categories and evaluate new alternatives. For example, research on brand extensions suggests that if the perceived fit between the extension and the parent brand is high (for example high similarity between the original and the extension product categories), consumers are likely to rely on the parent brand schema to evaluate the new alternative (Aaker and Keller 1990). Further research demonstrated that consumers not only take into account the similarity of product categories but also consider other factors included within brand schemas such as brand concept consistency (Park et al. 1991) and brand specific associations (Broniarczyk and Alba 1994a) in evaluating a new extension. Park et al. (1991) found that prestige brands are more extendible into categories with low feature similarity because consumers are likely to focus on prestige associations (versus feature similarity) in evaluating a new extension. Broniarczyk and Alba (1994a) showed that brand specific associations may dominate category similarity, particularly when knowledge of the brand is high.

Script is a schema about sequences of events in a period of time. For example, consumers may have scripts about shopping and paying for groceries, which involve sequences of events from entering into the store to paying at the checkout. Schemas and scripts are thought to be acquired over time based on experience and other sources (for example advertisements, other consumers, published information). Peracchio (1992) examined how young children acquire consumption-related scripts. She found that younger children were able to learn scripts as well as older children, when the materials were congruent with their encoding and retrieval abilities. Specifically, younger children's learning was enhanced by repetition and increasing the salience of the steps involved in the script.

Schema-based versus attribute-based processing

When do people rely on their schemas and when do they use individuating attribute information? Fiske and Neuberg (1990) suggest that people use a continuum of impression formation, ranging from category-based to more individuating processes. They propose that when you first meet a person, salient physical cues and labels are used for initial categorization. Once a person is categorized, schemas associated with the category are used for making judgements about the person. If perceivers are motivated, they may attempt to confirm this initial categorization. Category confirmation occurs when individuating information is consistent with schema-based expectations. Fiske and Neuberg (1990) suggest that initial confirmation may occur even when the individuating information is mixed (that is, both consistent and inconsistent) or irrelevant. Under these circumstances, people form judgements on the basis of their schema-based expectations because the evidence (for example individuating information) is not perceived strong enough to override schema-based expectations. However, if the individuating information is clearly inconsistent, perceivers are likely to re-categorize or subtype the target. If re-categorization is not successful, perceivers use individuating information to form their judgements.

Brewer (1988) suggests that perceivers automatically identify a person upon presentation. If the person is not relevant, no further processing takes place. However, if the person is relevant, personalization or categorization occurs depending on the level of involvement. Specifically, if the level of involvement is high, perceivers are likely to engage in bottom-up processing and rely on individuating attribute information to form their judgements (that is, personalization). In such a situation, category membership is stored as an attribute of the target in addition to other attributes. However, if the level of involvement is low, perceivers search for an appropriate category. If the features do not fully match the category schema, perceivers search among the subtypes of the category. Once an appropriate category or sub-category is found, further information processing is organized around that category.

Do consumers engage in category-based processing or are they likely to rely on the attributes of products in forming their judgements? Sujan (1985) showed that if the attribute information about a new product matches the features of an activated product category, category-based affective processes mediate consumers' judgements. However, if the attribute information does not match the features of an activated category, consumers' judgements are likely to be based on piecemeal processing of attribute information. Sujan (1985) also found that these effects were pronounced more for experts than novices. While novices relied on category-based processes regardless of discrepancy, experts were more likely to use attribute information when the information was discrepant from activated category schemas. These findings suggest that experts have well-developed schemas that enable them to process information about a new product more effectively than novices.

Product schemas include not only the attributes of a product, but usage occasions as well (for example cereal is associated with breakfast). Wansink and Ray (1996) examined how usage expansion advertising affects consumers' memory and attitudes. Consistent with Fiske and Neuberg's (1990) model, their findings indicate that schema-based processing, and consequently affect transfer, is likely to occur if proposed usage behaviour is mildly discrepant with existing behaviours. However, if proposed new uses are incongruent with existing behaviours, attribute-based processing is likely to occur. Although advertisements with incongruent behaviours are better remembered, they are generally evaluated less favourably.

Research indicates that consumers may have schemas about advertisements which are mostly exemplar based (Goodstein 1993). For example, a typical shampoo ad may feature a woman washing her hair. Goodstein (1993) demonstrated that television advertisements are processed in more detail when they are cosmetically atypical of the product category. He also found that typical ads could be processed in more detail when prior ad category affect increases. These findings can be interpreted using Brewer's (1988) model, which suggests that attribute-based processing is more likely under higher (versus lower) involvement. It is possible that affect-laden schemas are highly involving, leading to detailed processing when they are activated. Alternatively, activation of a certain schema may influence the extent of attribute-based processing. For example, Hong and Wyer (1989) found that country-of-origin information stimulated subjects to think more extensively about other product attribute information.

As noted earlier, experts' knowledge structures facilitate their understanding of information about new products in the same content domain. For example, when exposed to a continuous innovation (for example a new film-based camera), experts as compared to novices should have better comprehension. Consistent with this theorizing, Moreau et al. (2001a) found that experts report higher comprehension, more net benefits and higher preference for continuous innovations. However, experts' entrenched knowledge structures inhibit their understanding of information about discontinuous innovations or really new products (for example digital camera). This is because experts are likely to recognize discrepancies between a really new product (for example a digital camera) and existing products (for example film-based cameras). Consequently, they may be unsure of what knowledge can be transferred to the target. Moreau et al. (2001a) showed that experts' comprehension and appreciation of discontinuous innovations improved only when this entrenched knowledge is accompanied by relevant information from a supplementary knowledge base. These findings indicate that although well-developed schemas facilitate information processing in the same content domain (for example film-based cameras), they tend to impede information processing if experts can not engage in relation-based mapping from their knowledge domain to a new product (for example digital cameras).

Do consumers vary in the extent to which they engage in attribute-based and schema-based processing? Yoon (1997) examined age differences in consumers' processing strategies and found that older adults relied on schema-based processing particularly during their non-optimal part of the day. In addition, older adults exhibited greater use of attribute-based processing during their optimal part of the day when the information was discrepant from their schema-based expectations. These findings suggest that consumers are more likely to engage in schema-based processing when their ability to process information is lower (versus higher). Meyers-Levy and Maheswaran (1991) found that females are more likely to use a detailed processing strategy and males are more likely to use a schema-based strategy. However, these differences were eliminated when detailed attribute-based processing was encouraged by message characteristics (for example extreme cue incongruity) or response tasks (for example recall task). Their findings suggest that gender differences emerge because males elaborate ad claims less extensively than females, which produces differences in accessibility of ad claims.

Schema incongruity

Three types of processing responses – assimilation, **subtyping** and schema switching – are thought to occur when perceivers encounter instances with varying degrees of incongruity. If information about the new product is congruent with the schema, assimilation occurs (Sujan and Bettman 1989). Assimilation is the process by which a new concept is integrated into the schema. In other words, consumers utilize their prior knowledge associated with the category to evaluate the new product without making any changes in schema representation. Stayman et al. (1992) found that consumers who are exposed to an initial product-schema label and later received congruent information are likely to assimilate the information within the cued schema and base product-performance expectations on activated schema. Assimilation may also occur, when new information is slightly to moderately incongruent with schema-based expectations. If the schema is well developed, moderate incongruities are assimilated to schema representation by unique tags (O'Sullivan and Durso 1984; Sujan and Bettman 1989). Sujan and Bettman (1989) showed that schema plus tag model describe memory representation for a differentiated brand, which shares many consistent attributes with other brands in the category and has unique features that differentiates the brand.

If the information is highly incongruent with the existing schema and can not be filtered out, subtyping or schema switching is thought to occur. The subtyping process does not lead to a change in the general product category schema because subtyped members are set apart and considered unrepresentative of the category. Sujan and Bettman (1989) found that when a discrepant brand was subtyped, subjects recalled brand's distinguishing features better and fewer inferences were made about features not explicitly stated, suggesting that discrepant brand was set apart and categorized separately as a subtype. Stayman et al. (1992) showed that subjects who are exposed to an initial product-schema label and later received incongruent information are likely to discount the initial cue and switch to a second schema representation that is more consistent with attribute information. When subjects switched to a second schema, they based product-performance expectations on the second schema representation. Because both schema switching and subtyping can occur in response to incongruent information, future research is required to understand the conditions under which subtyping or switching occur.

The level of incongruity also influences consumers' search for information. Ozanne et al. (1992) examined how the level of incongruity influences breadth (that is, the number of different attributes searched) and depth (that is, search devoted to each attribute) of search behaviour during the categorization of new products. Their findings indicated that the breadth of search did not vary as a function of the level of incongruity. However, an inverted-U relationship was found between incongruity and depth of search. Specifically, subjects spent more time and effort processing information on a limited set of attributes when the information was moderately incongruent with their schema-based expectations.

How does schema incongruity influence product evaluations? Based on Mandler's (1982) hypothesis, Meyers-Levy and Tybout (1989) proposed that the level of congruity between a product and a more general schema may influence the nature of information processing and product evaluations. Specifically, Mandler (1982) argued that people prefer schema congruity because they like objects that confirm their expectations and allow predictability. However, congruent objects do not stimulate cognitive elaboration and consequently, positive responses that they generate are mild. In contrast, extreme incongruity leads to cognitive elaboration but such an elaboration may lead to frustration if it can not be resolved successfully. Moderate incongruities, on the other hand, are likely to generate positive affect because they generate cognitive elaboration, which leads to successful resolution of incongruity. In other words, Mandler (1982) proposed an inverted-U relationship between schema incongruity and product evaluations. While congruity and extreme incongruity are not likely to generate positive affect, moderate incongruity is likely to lead to more favourable evaluations.

Consistent with Mandler's (1982) propositions, Meyers-Levy and Tybout (1989) demonstrated that consumers, in particular non-dogmatics, had more favourable evaluations in response to moderate incongruity. Similarly, Stayman et al. (1992) found that consumers had more favourable evaluations when product-trial experiences were moderately incongruent with their pre-trial expectations as compared to congruity or extreme incongruity. Peracchio and Tybout (1996) extended these findings by examining the moderating effect of expertise on schema congruity effects. Experts are likely to know different types of products belonging to the category and can resolve any incongruity without much elaboration. However, novices (versus experts) will need to expand effort to resolve incongruity. Since cognitive elaboration and successful resolution of incongruity are presumed to generate positive affect, novices as compared to experts are more likely to experience schema congruity effects. Consistent with this theorizing, Peracchio and Tybout (1996) found that novices had more favourable evaluations in response to moderate incongruity (versus congruity or extreme incongruity). Expert consumers evaluations were unaffected by incongruity but influenced by product-specific associations.

Schema congruity effects were also tested in the context of consumers' responses to new products introduced by companies with established brand names. Meyers-Levy et al. (1994) found that consumers preferred products associated with moderately incongruent brand names (for example peanut-butter-flavoured cereal by Peter Pan) over products associated with congruent (for example peanut-butter-flavoured cereal by Kellogg) or incongruent brand names (for example peanut-butter-flavoured cereal by Frito-Lay). Although there is a considerable amount of consumer research that is supportive of

Mandler's (1982) theory, other research, particularly in the area of aesthetic responses, does not provide support. For example, Veryzer and Hutchinson (1998) examined the effects of prototypicality and unity on consumers' preference for design. Prototypicality refers to the degree to which an exemplar is representative of a category and can be varied by changing design parts in the domain of aesthetic responses. As the number of modified parts increases, prototypicality decreases in a linear fashion. Unity is a function of the relationship among different parts and has all-or-none character. Veryzer and Hutchinson manipulated unity and prototypicality by modifying line drawings of existing products. They found that as prototype distortion increased (that is, incongruity increased), consumers' aesthetic responses decreased, suggesting a linear relationship between congruity and aesthetic responses. They also showed that unity had a superadditive positive effect on aesthetic responses. The positive effects of unity and prototypicality were stronger when design variations were easily compared and visual properties were the only basis for judgement. Given that findings on aesthetic responses are different from those on product schemas, future research should compare the processes that underlie schema congruity effects in the context of aesthetic judgements and product evaluations.

The effect of accessibility of schemas on information processing and judgements

Knowledge can be activated or brought to mind only when it is present in memory. Availability refers to whether or not a knowledge structure is stored in memory. Once stored, a particular knowledge structure can be activated and may have an impact on judgements. The activation potential of stored knowledge has been referred to as accessibility (Higgins 1996). For example, if knowledge about country-of-origin is activated some time before the attribute information is presented, it affects the interpretation of information about specific attributes (Hong and Wyer 1990).

Product-related experiences (for example product usage or ownership) appear to be more accessible as compared to product-class information (Park et al. 1994). Because product-related experiences are more accessible, they influence consumers' assessment of subjective knowledge more than objective knowledge (for example product-class information). Park et al. (1994) suggest that the weak relationship between subjective knowledge (measured via self-report assessment of knowledge) and objective knowledge (measured via objective tests) can be explained in terms of greater accessibility of product-related experiences, which may 'underrepresent or misrepresent true knowledge about the domain' (Park et al. 1994: 79). Within product-related experiences, regularity and similarity influence the accessibility of the requisite information in memory (Menon 1993). In responding to behavioural frequency questions (for example 'How many boxes of cereal have you purchased in last six months?'), memory search was more extensive for irregular (versus regular) and dissimilar (versus similar) behaviours since such behaviours were less accessible (Menon 1993).

Research suggests that accessible schemas influence encoding and interpretation of incoming information. For example, country-of-origin information can sometimes be used as a stereotype and can influence product judgements (Hong and Wyer 1990; Maheswaran 1994). Maheswaran (1994) showed that when attribute information is unambiguous, experts based their evaluations on attribute information, whereas novices relied on country-of-origin, since they do not have extensive knowledge to understand attribute information. When the attribute information was ambiguous, experts used country-of-origin to selectively process and recall attribute information and novices used country-of-origin to interpret subsequent attribute information. These findings are consistent with research on stereotyping, which suggests that stereotypes bias information processing and judgement (for example Bodenhausen 1988).

Consumers' animosity toward a specific country can affect their purchase behaviour independent of their beliefs about the quality of products. Klein et al. (1998) showed that consumers who have high animosity toward a specific country do not buy products associated with that country although they think that products may be of high quality.

Accessibility of schemas depends on the frequency and recency of activation (Srull and Wyer 1979). For example, accessibility of a trait schema (for example hostile or polite) increases as perceivers encounter more schema-related behavioural concepts and when perceivers encounter schema-related behavioural concepts recently. Srull and Wyer (1979) showed that if accessibility of a trait schema increased due to frequency and recency of its activation, the likelihood that the accessible schema would be used to encode new information also increased. In addition, the effects of accessibility on trait judgements were much more pronounced when the encoded information was relatively ambiguous. Further research suggested that accessibility of alternative categories or constructs may attenuate the likelihood that the accessible schema would have an impact on judgement (Higgins et al. 1982). That is, the impact of an accessible schema increases if other concepts are not chronically more accessible. Also, accessible schemas are likely to influence encoding and judgements when they are relevant or applicable to the judgement at hand (Higgins 1996). Finally, the effect of accessible constructs on judgements decreases when perceivers become aware of the connection between accessibility and judgements (Martin et al. 1990).

Researchers have frequently used priming to manipulate accessibility of constructs. The priming procedure activates a stored knowledge unit, which increases its accessibility and consequently its effect on a subsequent judgement given that it is relevant and other concepts are not chronically accessible. For example, in Herr's (1989) experiments, subjects were primed with different price categories, ranging from extremely inexpensive to extremely expensive, and were asked to evaluate real and hypothetical car prices. When subjects were primed with moderately expensive or moderately inexpensive cars, their judgements of hypothetical car prices shifted toward the primed category (that is, assimilation effects). Moreover, these effects were pronounced more for consumers who were knowledgeable about cars, suggesting that priming effects depend on the existence of a category stored in memory. However, contrast effects were observed (that is, judgements shifted away from primed categories) when extremely inexpensive or expensive cars were primed. These findings, combined with similar finding in social psychology (for example Herr et al. 1983; Herr 1986), suggest that assimilation to the primed category occurs when category knowledge is available, primed category is not extreme, and ambiguous stimuli are judged. When extreme categories are primed, assimilation does not occur because the primed categories serve as a standard of comparison for judgements (Herr 1989).

It is possible to think of many other contexts that can serve as a prime and can influence consumer judgements. For example, when reading a magazine, the content of an article or an ad may influence the interpretation of subsequent ads. Yi (1990b) examined the effects of priming on the processing of ambiguous product information in advertisements. Subjects were first exposed to prime ads that emphasized either versatility or ease-of-use for a computer. After reading the prime ad, subjects were exposed to the target ad about a new brand of computer. Results showed that contextually primed attributes (that is, ease-of-use or versatility) were more accessible to consumers than unprimed attributes. More important, these variations influenced brand attitudes.

Television viewing affects consumers' perceptions of social reality by influencing encoding of information in a way that is more consistent with the content of television programming than social reality (Shrum et al. 1998). Shrum et al. (1998) found that heavy viewers of television formed beliefs that were more consistent with the content of TV programming as compared to light viewers. These findings indicate that accessibility of exemplars frequently portrayed on TV programmes are higher for heavy viewers (versus light viewers). Consequently, heavy viewers' judgements are more likely to be assimilated toward the content of TV programming as compared to judgements of light viewers. Shrum et al. (1998) showed that calling participants' attention to the relation between viewing frequency and their judgements eliminated assimilation effects because participants discounted the effect TV has as a source of information about social reality.

Research has shown that people exhibit self-positivity bias in estimating their risk of becoming ill (Perloff and Fetzer 1986). That is, people tend to underestimate their risk of becoming ill relative to others. Raghubir and Menon (1998) showed that increases in the accessibility of AIDS-related behaviours (for example listing the potential routes through which the HIV virus could be transmitted) increased the risk perceptions and reduced self-positivity biases. The ease of retrieval of AIDS-related information (high accessibility) at the time of processing an AIDS-related ad was found to improve effectiveness.

Consumers' perceptions of influence agents such as a salesperson are influenced by accessibility of ulterior motives. Campbell and Kirmani (2000) found that when a salesperson's behaviour increased the accessibility of a persuasion motive, that salesperson was perceived as less sincere regardless of cognitive capacity of the perceivers. In contrast, when an ulterior motive was less accessible, perceivers rated a salesperson as more sincere only when their cognitive capacity was constrained. These findings suggest that in order to apply persuasion knowledge, cognitive capacity is necessary unless ulterior motives are highly accessible.

Accessibility of category schemas depends on perceiver's processing goals and motivation (Brewer 1988; Fiske and Neuberg 1990). Perceivers are more likely to rely on schema-based expectations under low motivation. In contrast, under high motivation, when there are outcome dependency (Erber and Fiske 1984) and accountability instructions (Tetlock 1985), schema-based expectations are less salient and perceivers are more likely to rely on attributes of the individuals in forming judgements. Gürhan-Canli and Maheswaran (2000) found that when consumers use country-of-origin as a basis for judgement under low motivation or when the processing goal is to evaluate the country-of-origin, country-of-origin schemas are more accessible. Here, relevant evidence about the country-of-origin affects country-of-origin evaluations. However, if country-of-origin information is not highly accessible, such as under high motivation or if their processing goal directs their attention away from country-of-origin information, consumers are less likely to process attribute information about different products in relation to country-of-origin schemas.

As noted earlier, accessible schemas are likely to influence judgements when they are relevant to the judgement at hand. According to accessibility-diagnosticity model (Feldman and Lynch 1988), the likelihood that an input will be used as a basis for judgement is determined by (a) the accessibility of the input, (b) the accessibility of other inputs, and (c) the perceived diagnosticity of the input for judgements. For example, when consumers were asked to report behavioural frequency judgements, their responses depended on the accessibility and diagnosticity of memory-based information (for example rate of occurrence) and context-based information (for example response alternatives provided in the survey) (Menon et al. 1995). Because regular (versus irregular) behaviours were highly accessible and diagnostic, frequency judgements for regular behaviours were not influenced by variations in response alternatives. However, because irregular behaviours were not highly accessible, frequency judgements for irregular behaviours were influenced by the frequencies presented in the response alternatives (Menon et al. 1995).

Herr et al. (1991) found that word-of-mouth information had a disproportionate impact on judgements because of its accessibility. The effect of word-of-mouth was reduced when more diagnostic information (for example prior impressions or extremely negative information) was accessible. Aaker (2000) examined the extent to which accessibility and diagnosticity of associations embedded in persuasion appeals better account for the cross-cultural differences. When subjects were prompted to elaborate, accessibility of the associations increased and differences between cultures were eliminated, providing more support for differential accessibility of culture-relevant constructs. That is, distinct cultural associations may be valued in another culture but do not generally impact consumer judgements in non-target cultures because of their lower accessibility at an individual level.

Ahluwalia and Gürhan-Canli (2000) showed that accessibility of extension information moderates the effects of information valence and category similarity on brand evaluations. On the basis of accessibility-diagnosticity model, it was proposed that as the accessibility of extension information increases, so does its likelihood with which it will be used for evaluating the family brand. Consistent with this theorizing, Ahluwalia and Gürhan-Canli (2000) found that under higher accessibility, negative information about the extension led to dilution and positive information led to enhancement of the family brand regardless of extension category (that is, far or close). In contrast, under lower accessibility, the effect of extension information was based on its diagnosticity.

So far, we have discussed situational accessibility of schemas due to recency and frequency of activation. Schemas also exert impact on judgements when they are chronically accessible (Higgins et al. 1982). Chronic accessibility results from persistent differences in what is primed by one's typical situations (Fiske and Taylor 1991). If a personality dimension is typically accessible to a person (for example friendly), that person is more likely to remember and describe others in terms of how friendly they are (Higgins et al. 1982). These types of traits are defined as schematic traits and are descriptive of and very important to people. In a series of experiments, Aaker and Lee (2001) showed that more elaborate processing occurs when information is compatible (versus incompatible) with one's self-schema. Specifically, they found that consumers with highly accessible independent self-views were more likely to elaborate on and be persuaded by the information with a promotion focus (for example enjoyment). In contrast, consumers with highly accessible interdependent self-views were more likely to elaborate on and be persuaded by the information with a prevention focus (for example safety). Aaker (1999) showed that both schematic and situationally accessible traits influence attitudes toward a brand, based on its personality associations. For example, more favourable attitudes on the excitement dimension were obtained for low versus high self-monitoring subjects when excitement was a schematic trait. In contrast, more favourable attitudes on the excitement dimension were obtained for high versus low self-monitors when excitement was situationally accessible.

Schema change

We have noted that when exposed to schema incongruent information, perceivers may consider incongruent instances as exceptions and form subtypes within the category. When incongruent instances are subtyped, incongruent attributes are stored separately and consequently, do not lead to a change in the content of the schema. This model has been referred to as the subtyping model and suggests that schema change is less likely when instances are extremely incongruent. In contrast, schema change is expected, when subtypes can not be formed (for example when the typicality of instances increases). Weber and Crocker (1983) proposed two other models to account for the modification of schemas in response to incongruent information. The **bookkeeping model** posits that each piece of new information leads to an incremental modification of the schema and schema change occurs over time as perceivers are exposed to more incongruent information. The **conversion model** posits that schemas change when exposed to extremely atypical instances. As typicality of an instance increases, less schema change is expected. In Weber and Crocker's study incongruent information was either condensed in describing a few group members, or dispersed across several group members. In the *condensed* condition, a small subset of group members displayed all incongruent behaviours. In the *dispersed* condition, incongruent information was distributed across all members so that each one displayed one incongruent behaviour. Since only one incongruent behaviour was featured for each member, each would be perceived as relatively high in typicality. In contrast, condensed information depicted a few instances that featured several incongruent attributes. Such instances would be perceived as low in typicality. Weber and Crocker (1983) found that, consistent with the subtyping model, when incongruent information is condensed in a few instances, perceivers subtype these instances and schemas do not change. Their findings were also consistent with the bookkeeping model. As the amount of incongruent information increased, more schema change was observed. Further research in this area provided evidence consistent with the subtyping model (for example Johnston and Hewstone 1992; Hewstone et al. 1994). Some support for the conversion model was found when the group was perceived as homogeneous (Hewstone et al. 1992).

Extant research on dilution and enhancement of brand names has produced findings that are consistent with both subtyping and bookkeeping. Romeo (1991) reported marginally significant findings, which seem to be consistent with the subtyping model. Dilution effects were observed only when incongruent information pertained to a typical (versus atypical) extension. In Keller and Aaker's (1992) study, consistent with subtyping, an average quality brand was evaluated more favourably when the company was successful in extending to relatively similar but distinct product types (that is, high typicality). In Loken and John's (1993) study, when beliefs were measured first, consistent with bookkeeping, dilution effects were found regardless of the typicality of the extension. Interestingly, when typicality judgements were made salient, subtyping may have occurred, because extremely incongruent description did not lead to a change in prior beliefs. Park and colleagues (Park et al. 1993; Milberg et al. 1997) also found support for both models in studies that examined the effects of sub-branding (that is, a new brand name used in combination with the existing family brand name) and direct brand extension strategies. Consistent with bookkeeping, when a direct extension strategy was used, the target brands were evaluated less favourably regardless of typicality. However, consistent with subtyping, the use of sub-branding reduced dilution effects. When consumers were provided a basis (for example sub-branding) for separating atypical extension from the brand name, negative feedback effects were minimized.

The observation that brand name dilution and enhancement can be guided by either the subtyping or the bookkeeping model seems to suggest that consumers' use of these models is moderated by other factors. Gürhan-Canli and Maheswaran (1998) showed that processing motivation is likely to influence the process by which brand schemas are modified. Under low motivation, consumers are less likely to expend the effort to process the attribute information in detail and are likely to engage in category-based processing. In response to incongruent information, consumers are expected to use the subtyping model, since it requires less effort to add to a schema by forming subtypes than to revise it. That is, the formation of subtypes would resolve incongruency without effortful attribute processing. Under high motivation, consumers are expected to process all information that is available to them. In other words, consumers are likely to expend effort to process information piecemeal as in bookkeeping, since this model suggests that all information is processed regardless of typicality of instances, each piece of new information contributing to schema modification. Consistent with this theorizing, Gürhan-Canli and Maheswaran (1998) found that brand schemas changed regardless of typicality of instances under high motivation. In contrast, under low motivation, extremely incongruent instances were subtyped and did not lead to a change in brand schema.

Summary

Consumers' knowledge content is represented by a set of associations linked in schemas and scripts. We reviewed research that examined when and how such knowledge structures influence consumer judgements and how incongruent information is processed. Next, we discuss how consumers retain and retrieve knowledge in memory.

Memory

It is well known that consumers have poor memories for brand names, attribute information, prices and advertising (Keller 1987; Meyers-Levy 1989b;

Morwitz et al. 1998). For example, Block and Morwitz (1999) showed that consumers frequently used shopping lists for grocery shopping as an external memory aid. How can consumers' memory performance be improved? What are the factors that influence the processes that underlie memory performance? We review research that examines the processes by which information is stored in and retrieved from memory. We also briefly discuss research on the relationship between memory processes and consumer judgements.

The classic memory model proposed by Atkinson and Shiffrin (1968) suggests that there are three distinct but interrelated memory systems: **sensory memory, short-term memory** and **long-term memory**. Sensory memory is temporary storage of the information received from senses. If the information is retained, it is transferred to short-term memory. Short-term memory has a limited capacity and holds the information that individuals are currently processing. Long-term memory is the system for retaining information for a long time. Information is transferred from short-term memory to long-term memory, if individuals think about the meaning of a stimulus and relate it to other information in memory. In other words, if processing resources are sufficient at the encoding stage, knowledge can be integrated with what is already available in memory and retrieved in the future. Although experimental research does not consistently support the distinction between short-term and long-term memories, many contemporary cognitive theories utilize this distinction (Matlin 1998).

Network models (for example associative network model, ACT model, parallel distributed processing approach) suggest that long-term memory can be represented as a network of nodes and connecting links (Collins and Loftus 1975; Anderson 1983; Masson 1995). Nodes represent specific information (for example brands, attributes, evaluations, product category information), which are connected to each other via links on the basis of some set of relationships. If one node is activated, other nodes associated with it also become triggered (that is, spreading activation: Collins and Loftus 1975). The strength of the associations among different nodes determines which nodes will be activated.

Consumer memory for advertising

Exposure to advertising forms different types of nodes in long-term memory. These nodes may represent brand-specific information, ad-specific-information, brand identification, product category, and evaluative reactions (Hutchinson and Moore 1984). Consumer goals (for example brand ad evaluation) at the encoding stage influence the degree to which ad-specific versus brand-specific nodes are formed. While ad-specific nodes can be formed under both brand evaluation and ad evaluation goals, more brand-specific nodes can be formed under brand (versus ad) evaluation goal. Moreover, when consumers focus on brand specific information under brand evaluation goals, stronger links are expected between the brand name and other nodes.

Consumers' memory for brand-related information can be improved if retrieval cues are present when consumers are asked to recall brand-related information (Keller 1987). Ad retrieval cues such as verbal or visual information contained in ads activate relevant nodes in memory via the process of spreading activation and increase the likelihood that brand-specific information will be retrieved.

According to the **encoding specificity principle** (Tulving 1974), retrieval cues improve memory performance only when they are specifically encoded with the target information. Consistent with this principle, Keller (1991a) found that, compared to a no-additional-cue control group, subjects recalled greater numbers of ad-related (brand-related) cognitive responses with an ad execution (brand claims) cue. In addition, retrieval cues were found to inhibit the recall of less strongly associated information in memory. Compared to a no-additional-cue control group, subjects recalled fewer ad-related (brand-related) cognitive responses with a brand claims (ad execution) cue.

Costley et al. (1997) found that presentation medium influenced retrieval cue effectiveness. Specifically, they found that consumers were more likely to recall a visual stimulus than an auditory stimulus when visual retrieval cues were used. Similar findings were obtained for the auditory stimulus, when subjects were under lower imaging condition. These findings are consistent with the encoding specificity principle and suggest that matching of presentation medium with an execution cue may improve memory performance.

Consumers' memory performance can be reduced as a function of learning additional related information because such information creates a greater number of links to a node. As the number of links increases, the probability of retrieving any particular link decreases. This has been referred to as interference effects (Tulving and Psotka 1971). Proactive (retroactive) interference effects occur because of material that has been learned before (after) the target is encountered. Burke and Srull (1988) found evidence for **proactive interference** and **retroactive interference** effects due to exposure to ads for other products of the same manufacturer and for competing brands in the same product class. Repetition did not improve memory performance when there was competitive interference. Further research examined the moderating effect of ad valence on memory performance in the context of competitive interference (Keller 1991b). A laboratory experiment suggested that when the level of competitive advertising was low (for example one competing ad) recall of brand claims was lower when competing ads differed in valence (for example good target ad and bad competing ad). However, the presence of a competing ad did not interfere with retrieval of cognitive responses or evaluations of the target brand. When the level of competitive advertising was high and the ads varied in valence, subjects had difficulty retrieving evaluations of the target brand.

How can the effects of competitive interference be reduced? Keller (1987) found that the effect of interference can be reduced by providing retrieval cues. Varying the ad context can reduce the competitive interference effects by increasing the number of contextual cues for retrieval (Unnava and Sirdeshmukh 1994). Based on the encoding variability hypothesis (Melton 1970), Unnava and Sirdeshmukh (1994) argued that the use of varying ad executions or changing the modality of the target advertising help reduce competitive interference effects better than repeating the same execution or repeating the ad in the same modality, respectively. The encoding variability hypothesis suggests that the context in which the target is embedded forms part of the memory trace for that target. Because contextual information can act as retrieval cues, presenting the target in varied contexts can improve retrieval by providing multiple contextual cues. However, contextual cues can cause interference effects if ads for competing products and the target product share similar contextual factors (Kumar 2000).

Kent and Allen (1994) demonstrated that competitive interference effects were reduced when familiar brand names were used. Specifically, when subjects were exposed to ads for familiar brands, no interference effects were observed in the presence of competitive ads for familiar and unfamiliar brands. Consumers have established schemas for familiar brands with stronger links among the product class, brand and its attributes. New attribute information learned through advertising is likely to be organized by brand under product class. However, for unfamiliar brands, new nodes would be created under the product class linking attribute information to these new brands. When the product class is activated, it will be easier to retrieve attribute information about the familiar (versus unfamiliar) brand because attribute information will be linked only to the node of the relevant brand.

While research reveals evidence for competitive interference effects particularly for unfamiliar brands (for example Keller 1987; Burke and Srull 1988; Kent and Allen 1994; Unnava and Sirdeshmukh 1994), other research shows that advertising clutter may not significantly affect consumers' ability to remember brand names (Brown and Rothschild 1993). It is important to note that in Brown and Rothschild's (1993) experiments, subjects were exposed to ads for brands in different product categories. It is possible that interference effects increase when advertised products are in the same (versus different) product categories.

Consumers' recall of message content also varies as a function of level of subjective comprehension. Mick (1992) distinguishes between message-based surface-level comprehension and receiver-based deeper levels of comprehension. Surface-level comprehension involves meanings related to or inferences derived from explicit message content. In contrast, receiver-based comprehension involves inferences derived from general product or situational knowledge and meanings related to personalized embellishments derived from self-experiences. Mick (1992) found that deeper levels of comprehension were associated with improved delayed message recall. Interestingly, at deeper levels of comprehension, message recall decreased, indicating that self-related associations inhibit the recall of advertising messages.

How do pictorial and verbal components of an ad influence memory processes? When consumers are exposed to ad copy (that is, words), verbal codes are formed in memory. However, when they are exposed to pictures, visual or imaginal codes are created. The dual coding model suggests that memory performance may improve when pictures (versus words) are used because it is easier for consumers to form verbal codes for pictures as compared to forming visual codes for words (Paivio 1986). Therefore, pictures (versus words) can be retrieved more easily since they are associated with alternative retrieval routes in memory. Childers and Houston (1984) found that, when processing was directed at appearance features, picture superiority occurred in both immediate and delayed recall tasks. However, when processing was directed at the semantic content of the advertisements, picture superiority occurred only in delayed recall tasks. Macklin (1994) examined the effect of dual coding on children's product-related recall. She found that dual coding (that is, when visuals overlapped the audio information) was very effective in improving memory performance of younger (that is, pre-schoolers) and older (that is, school-age) children. The effect was particularly pronounced for younger children, who could not successfully recall product-related information when partial visuals (for example visuals that omitted the brand character or the target product) were used. Unnava and Burnkrant (1991a) showed that when verbal information in an ad encourages imagery, picture superiority effects are reduced. Specifically, they found that pictures that exemplify verbal information in an ad improved retrieval only when words were not imagery-provoking.

Considerable amount of research examined how the congruity among different parts of an ad (for example copy, picture, brand name) influences recall and judgements. Lutz and Lutz (1977) showed that ads that integrated the brand name and the picture (for example picture depicted the meaning of the brand) were remembered better than ads that did not integrate the brand and the picture. Edell and Staelin (1983) found that recall for brand-related information improved when pictures and copy contained the same information as compared to a picture only condition. Schmitt et al. (1993) suggest that congruity of different elements in ads leads to improvement in retrieval processes because nodes are more closely associated if the information represented is related. That is, stronger links are likely to be formed among different nodes when the brand name, picture and copy convey similar (versus dissimilar) information. Consistent with this theorizing, Schmitt et al. (1993) found that ads containing relations among different ad components were remembered better than ads that have unrelated ad components. While there is some convergent evidence supporting the effectiveness of integrated ad parts, other studies suggest that incongruent elements in advertising may lead to superior recall (Houston et al. 1987; Heckler and Childers 1992).

Heckler and Childers (1992) proposed that incongruency has two dimensions: relevancy and expectancy. Relevancy refers to the extent to which different pieces of information convey the same theme. In advertising, relevancy is high if picture and copy convey information about the same attribute. Expectancy refers to the degree to which the information is consistent with an overall schema. In advertising, expectancy is high if picture-based expectancies are confirmed in the copy. Heckler and Childers (1992) found that unexpected (versus expected) information was recalled more easily because it was encoded in detail. Relevant (versus irrelevant) information was recalled more easily but this effect was not due to detailed encoding. In general, the results suggest that unexpected information as compared to expected information leads to improved memory performance, particularly for recall of brand names and product categories. Memory performance also improves if information conveyed via different elements of an ad are integrated and perceived to be relevant (versus irrelevant).

Consumer memory for brand names

As noted earlier, a brand name's memorability may be inhibited as the number of associations linked to a brand name increases due to interference effects. It is also possible to argue the opposite to the extent that these associations can act as retrieval cues. According to the encoding variability hypothesis (Melton 1970), concepts are encoded with their contexts. When the same information is presented in varied contexts, multiple routes are formed in memory, which are associated with the same information. Because contextual cues can act as retrieval cues, identical information presented in varied contexts should be better remembered than the same information repeated in the same context. Consistent with this theorizing, Unnava and Burnkrant (1991b) found that memory for a fictitious brand name improved when varied ad executions were used (versus same ad execution repeated). Meyers-Levy (1989b) found that the distinctiveness of the brand name moderated the effect of association set size on brand memory. For distinctive brand names (for example low frequency words), the number of associations linked to a brand name did not have any effect on brand name memory because such brands elicit distinctive processing. For non-distinctive brand names (for example high frequency), memory performance improved with small rather than large association sets.

A brand's association with its category can be enhanced by increasing consumers' motivation to categorize the brand. Fazio et al. (1992b) found that stronger associations between the product category and the brand were formed if the brand was not identified until the end of the ad as in the case of mystery ads. When consumers are exposed to mystery ads, they want to find out what is being advertised and consequently are highly attentive to the brand's category.

One study identified positive mood as another factor that enhances the association between a brand name and its category (Lee and Sternthal 1999). Specifically, positive mood as compared to neutral mood fosters relational processing on the basis of category membership (Isen et al. 1992). Consequently, brand-name retrieval is enhanced when product category is used as a retrieval cue. Positive mood can also enhance brand rehearsal as part of the categorization process. Positive mood subjects are more likely to engage in relational elaboration, which induces a focus on brand names and leads to more rehearsal as compared to the neutral mood condition.

The strength of association between a brand name and different product categories may influence brand extension evaluations through its impact on retrieval processes (Dawar 1996; Herr et al. 1996). Dawar (1996) showed that for brands strongly associated with a single product, retrieval inhibition effects reduced the activation of different product associations, lowering the perceptions of fit between new extensions and the brand. However, for brands that are strongly associated with multiple products, retrieval of different associations influence perceptions of fit. Herr et al. (1996) suggest that a brand's association with a category can be differentiated on the basis of its directional association. For example, category dominance is the strength of the category to brand associations (that is, the extent to which category label activates the brand). Herr et al. (1996) found that consumers' recall of a proposed extension is greater for category dominant versus weaker brands and for closely versus distantly related target categories. Subsequent research suggested that accessibility of nondominant brands may increase when they introduce high fit brand extensions (Morrin 1999). Introduction of high fit extensions enhances the association between the brand and the category, resulting in improved brand retrieval.

What are the different types of processes that consumers use when they attempt to retrieve brand names after they have encoded brand names as a result of being exposed to various promotions (for example ads, sponsorships) or other informational sources (for example word-of-mouth, *Consumer Reports*)? As noted earlier, cued retrieval is likely to be the dominant process particularly when brand name and message content are strongly encoded (Keller 1991a). Research indicates that when cued retrieval fails, consumers are likely to utilize different processes depending on their level of motivation (Pham and Johar 1997). When cued retrieval fails, consumers are thought to rely on memory-trace refreshment if motivation for accuracy is high and trace is accessible and diagnostic. Theoretical frameworks on memory suggest that the perceptual and contextual details are often instrumental in revealing the sources of memory (Johnson et al. 1993). For example, in the context of advertising consumers may attempt to retrieve some perceptual and contextual details of the ads, which are subsequently utilized to retrieve the brand name. This process is effortful as it entails 'an attempt to revive (bring to consciousness) the original learning episode with its perceptual and contextual details' (Pham and Johar 1997: 251). If memory-trace refreshment fails (because it is either inaccessible or not diagnostic), consumers are thought to rely on schematic inferences. Schematic inferencing entails the use of a general schema to identify the brand, indicating that a brand name is likely to be retrieved to the extent that it is consistent with an evoked schema. For example, Johar and Pham (1999) found that sponsor identification is biased toward brands that are prominent in the marketplace and semantically related to the event. In other words, consumers use prominence and relatedness as heuristic cues in identifying the brands that are likely to sponsor an event. Pham and Johar (1997) suggest that consumers are likely to use pure guessing only as a last resort, only if other processes fail and there is little motivation to retrieve the brand name.

The effect of memory on judgements

What is the relationship between memory and judgements? Hastie and Park (1986) propose that the relationship between memory and judgements depends on whether a judgement is formed while the information is being presented (that is, online) or judgement is formed based on the information retrieved from memory. If perceivers form their judgements online, they are likely to retrieve that judgement when they are asked to express their opinion. However, if they have not formed judgements online, their judgements would depend on the information they can retrieve from memory. When the information is processed online, the first few pieces of information are particularly important in forming evaluations, leading to primacy effects (Hastie and Park 1986). In addition, online information processing encourages more integrative processing, resulting in many associative links between the target and information and better recall of information (Srull and Wyer 1989). When judgements are memory-based, perceivers have better memory for recently encountered information and recently acquired information has a disproportionate impact on evaluations (Hastie and Park 1986; Srull and Wyer 1989). Since perceivers do not try to integrate information at the time of presentation, there will be fewer associative links between the target and the behavioural information, resulting in poorer recall of information. Also, because perceivers' judgements will depend on the information retrieved, there should be a correlation between recall and judgements (Hastie and Park 1986; Herr et al. 1991; Park and Hastak 1994).

Park and Hastak (1994) investigated how involvement at encoding and at judgement influence the processes mediating memory-based judgements. When involvement was low at the time of memory-based judgement, subjects simply retrieved their prior evaluations. However, when involvement was higher at the time of judgement than at the time of encoding, subjects recalled and used specific product information in forming their judgements. These findings suggest that involvement at the time of judgement increases the intensity of search for judgement-relevant information.

Consumers' autobiographical memories were found to affect product judgements when a marketing stimuli (for example an ad) evokes affect-laden memories and when the marketing stimuli establishes a link between autobiographical memories and the target product (Sujan et al. 1993). Sujan et al. (1993) showed that when autobiographical memories are prompted brand evaluations did not vary as a function of argument strength, indicating that the brand evaluations were not based on attribute information but were based on affect associated with evoked memory.

Research suggests that consumers' recall of product-related experiences can be influenced by marketing communications (Braun 1999). In a series of experiments, subjects first tasted the target product and half of the subjects were subsequently exposed to advertisements about the target product. Subjects who were exposed to the advertisements reported product experiences that were consistent with the implications of these advertisements (Braun 1999). These findings suggest that retrieval of product-related experiences can be distorted by information acquired after consumption.

While previous research highlights the important role of ad or product involvement in forming related memory traces, Hawkins and Hoch (1992) showed that consumers' memory for trivia statements can influence their belief in such statements under very low levels of involvement. Familiarity was found to mediate the effect of memory on truth ratings. Consumers rated trivia statements as more true when they were exposed to these statements before and the effect increased when the statements were repeated. Subsequent research suggested that elderly are more prone to such repetition effects due to age-related deficits in memory (Law et al. 1998). However, when memory was enhanced via an imagery task during encoding, the difference between older and younger subjects was eliminated.

In summary, research on memory processes focused on understanding consumer memory for advertising and brand names. Recent research has also highlighted the important role of memory on consumer decision making. Next, we investigate consumer inferences on the basis of available information and how consumers search for more information.

Inferences and information search

Consumers make inferences about the quality of a product or service on the basis of available intrinsic and extrinsic cues (Szybillo and Jacoby 1974). For example, consumers may infer lower quality from lower prices (Rao and Monroe 1989), higher quality from higher advertising costs (Kirmani 1990) and higher reliability from longer warranties (Broniarczyk and Alba 1994b). As discussed earlier, consumers also utilize brand names and country-of-origin information to infer the quality of new products (for example Aaker and Keller 1990; Maheswaran 1994). Research suggests that consumers infer value from irrelevant but unique attributes particularly when the product is priced toward the top end of all alternatives (Carpenter et al. 1994). When the price is high, consumers infer that the unique attribute is valuable even though they may be explicitly told that this attribute is irrelevant. Consumers are less likely to draw such inferences from irrelevant attributes when the price is low indicating little additional value.

Consumers draw inferences about marketers' motives on the basis of information about product performance, prices, promotions or advertising. Such inferences were found to mediate consumers' attitudes toward products and purchase intentions (Folkes 1984, 1988; Bitner 1990; Taylor 1994; Tripp et al. 1994; Brown and Dacin 1997; Campbell 1999; Raghubir and Corfman 1999; Dawar and Pillutla 2000; Sen et al. 2001). Most research in this area utilized an attributional approach to understand how consumers arrive at inferences regarding marketers' motives (Folkes 1988). For example, Folkes (1984) found that stability (that is, temporary or permanent) and locus of product failure (that is, consumer or manufacturer) influenced expectancies for future product failures and consequently preference for a refund as opposed to an exchange. Firm-related causes and controllability were also significantly related with anger and desire to hurt business. Similarly, in a service delay context, Taylor (1994) found that perceived service provider control over a delay resulted in greater anger. In general, understanding the customer's attribution processes and providing customers with logical explanations and compensations can mitigate dissatisfaction in the context of product failure (Bitner 1990). Research suggests that a company's response (for example unambiguous support, ambiguous support, stonewalling) interact with consumers' prior perceptions of the brand to determine brand attitudes in the context of a product-harm crisis (Dawar and Pillutla 2000). When consumers have weak expectations about the brand, post crisis brand attitudes were significantly lower in both the stonewalling and ambiguous response cases. In contrast, there was no negative effect of product-harm crisis if the company provided unambiguous support. In addition, there was no decline in brand equity when prior expectations were strong and the response was ambiguous. These findings underscore the important role of prior expectations in drawing inferences in the context of product failures.

Raghubir and Corfman (1999) used an attributional framework to understand the effect of price promotions on pre-trial brand evaluations. They found that consistency with past promotional behaviour and distinctiveness of promotions in terms of how common it is to promote in the industry affect evaluations. Consumers had more negative evaluations when the brand has not been promoted previously and when promotions are uncommon in the industry. Furthermore, novices were more likely to use promotions to infer product quality. Consumers generate inferences regarding a company's motive not only when price promotions are used to reduce prices but also when the company decides to increase prices. Campbell (1999) showed that when consumers inferred a negative motive for a price increase, the price increase was evaluated less fair and perceived unfairness mediated the effect of price increase on shopping intentions. Company's reputation moderated this effect such that consumers were less likely to infer a bad motive if the firm had a good reputation. Sen et al. (2001) found that consumers were likely to boycott a company in response to an unjustifiable price increase if they inferred that the boycott would be successful and they did not expect to incur much cost to boycott.

Attributional framework has also been applied to understanding consumer inferences from advertising. For example, Pechmann (1992) showed that two-sided ads (that is, ads that provide both positive and negative information) were effective when negatively correlated (versus uncorrelated) attributes were used. Correlational inferences as well as inferences about the advertiser's honesty (that is, correspondent inferences) improved overall brand evaluations. Tripp et al. (1994) found that, if celebrities endorse multiple products, consumers perceptions of expertise and liking of the celebrity decrease via attributions of trust. Consumers' resistance to persuasive attempts can also be examined within an attributional framework. For example, Rose et al. (1992) found a significant relationship between subjects' attributional thinking and conformity in the context of resistance to peer pressure to use drugs and alcohol. Specifically, conformity to group pressure was reduced when subjects engaged in attributional thinking concerning the group's behaviour and made external (versus internal) attributions. As also noted by Weiner (2000), future research can utilize attributional framework to investigate consumers inferences regarding marketers' motives. Although some research has focused on understanding consumers' inferences concerning product and promotion related motives, relatively little research has examined the effect of non-product associations (for example corporate social responsibility) on inferences and brand equity (Brown and Dacin 1997; Folkes and Kamins 1999).

Inferences based on incomplete information

Consumers often make judgements about products or services on the basis of incomplete information. Kardes (1993) suggests that consumers respond to incomplete information in three different ways. They ignore incomplete information, draw inferences about missing values or search for more information. When do consumers ignore incomplete information and when do they generate inferences on the basis of available information? Inferences can be generated spontaneously when inferential cues are salient to consumers at the time of decision making (Dick et al. 1990; Broniarczyk and Alba 1994b). In particular, consumers use intuitive theories about the relationships between attributes to a greater extent than other salient cues in making inferences (Broniarczyk and Alba 1994b). Another factor that moderates inference generation is level of expertise. Specifically, experts as compared to novices are more likely to detect omissions and adjust their evaluations for missing attributes (Sanbonmatsu et al. 1992). In addition, Sanbonmatsu et al. (1991) showed that novices' (versus experts') inferences about unknown attributes can become more extreme over time when perceivers do not remember the absence of information.

Research also suggests that consumers are more likely to generate spontaneous inferences from implicit conclusions when involvement or need for cognition is high versus low (Kardes 1988; Stayman and Kardes 1992). Moreover, self-generated inferences (versus explicit conclusions) can lead to more favourable and accessible brand attitudes, particularly for people who are more responsive to internal cues (that is, low self-monitors: Stayman and Kardes 1992). Research demonstrates that consumers miscomprehend advertising claims to a large extent and consequently draw invalid inferences (Jacoby and Hoyer 1987). Johar (1995) showed that the possibility of drawing invalid inferences from advertising claims varies as a function of involvement and type of claim. She found that consumers were more likely to draw invalid inferences from incomplete comparisons (that is, comparisons that do not name a referent) at the time of processing under higher (versus lower) involvement. In contrast, only less involved consumers were found to be deceived from inconspicuous qualification claims (that is, parenthetical qualifying information that limits the scope of a claim), because such claims require detailed processing of ads for non-deception. Disclosures to correct invalid inferences are used only under high motivation and ability conditions (Johar and Simmons 2000).

When consumers recognize missing attributes, they generally form less extreme evaluations (Huber and McCann 1982; Johnson and Levin 1985). Less extreme evaluations result because consumers may (a) infer neutral values for missing information, (b) adjust evaluations to compensate for uncertainty or (c) treat missing information as a negative cue (Huber and McCann 1982; Yamagishi and Hill 1983; Simmons and Lynch 1991). While less extreme evaluations may be obtained due to inferential processes, subsequent research found that reduced attention to attribute information may lead to less extreme evaluations when incomplete values are presented in the context of competitive information (Simmons and Lynch 1991). The experimental data reported by Simmons and Lynch (1991) indicated lower levels of inference making and provided support for the notion that inferences will be made when consumers are sufficiently motivated (Kardes 1988) and when an inference rule is accessible in memory and perceived to be diagnostic (Dick et al. 1990).

Information search

Research suggests that consumers search for more information to reduce their uncertainty prior to purchase (Urbany et al. 1989; Jacoby et al. 1994). Jacoby et al. (1994) examined how choice uncertainty is reduced as a function of information acquisition. They found that as consumers search for more information their uncertainty is reduced in a linear or in an accelerating fashion in an environment characterized by multiple options (for example alternative brands) and properties (for example several attributes). Accelerating uncertainty reduction is particularly dominant when consumers engage in within-options, across-properties searches. In other words, when consumers look at different properties of an option before searching for information for another option, reductions in uncertainty are observed later in the process when some information is available for all options. In contrast, when consumers engage in across-options, within-properties searches, substantial reductions in uncertainty are observed early in the process since some information about each option is obtained relatively earlier.

Urbany et al. (1989) distinguished between two types of uncertainty: knowledge and search uncertainty. Knowledge uncertainty refers to uncertainty regarding information about alternatives and search uncertainty refers to uncertainty regarding which alternative to choose. While choice uncertainty is correlated positively with search, knowledge uncertainty has a negative effect on search behaviour (Urbany et al. 1989). These findings are consistent with previous research, which suggests that objective knowledge facilitates asking of attribute questions and is associated with seeking information about a greater number of attributes (Brucks 1985). Moreover, objective knowledge improves search efficiency and reduces seeking information about inappropriate alternatives.

Prior knowledge influences not only the amount of information search but also the order of information acquisition. Simonson et al. (1988) found that information is acquired earlier when prior beliefs about the attribute values are uncertain and less favourable. Research also suggests that consumers follow information search patterns that are consistent with prior beliefs. For example, John et al. (1986) found that subjects who strongly believe in a positive price–quality relationship sample only higher priced products and those without such strong beliefs engage in more random sampling.

Prior knowledge influences search through its impact on consumers' ability to ask for relevant information. Research suggests that age is another factor that affects consumers' ability to search for information (Cole and Balasubramanian 1993; Gregan-Paxton and John 1997). Elderly compared to younger subjects are less likely to search intensely and to select an appropriate product particularly when choices are memory based. Such age differences are eliminated when subjects are asked to write information down (Cole and Balasubramanian 1993). Age differences were also observed in a study which investigated children's adaptivity to complex decision-making environments (Gregan-Paxton and John 1997). Older children adapted to complex environments by reducing search effort. Younger children reduced their search effort only when substantial search costs are made salient.

While previous research focused on ability related factors in influencing search process, relatively little research examined the effect of motivational factors on search behaviour. Lee et al. (1999) explored the effect of accountability and issue involvement on information acquisition. They found that accountability increases search effort regardless of level of prior knowledge, whereas issue involvement increases search effort only when prior knowledge is low. These findings suggest that motivational factors interact with consumers' prior knowledge to influence information search. Future research is required to address how ability and motivation-related factors jointly determine search. Moreover, the internet has become an important source of information for consumers.

In summary, we see that consumers make inferences about product quality and marketers' motives using external and internal cues, particularly when ability or motivation is high and when inference rules are accessible and diagnostic. Consumers search for more information to reduce uncertainty. Research also suggests that prior knowledge influences information search.

Conclusion

We have examined how consumers attend to, perceive, categorize, retrieve and utilize market-related information. Cognitive processes that underlie consumer evaluations and behaviour have been a vibrant research area with much focus on category accessibility and use of category knowledge, memory processes and information search. We reviewed work in this area and identified research opportunities.

Notes

1 It is important to note that different models have been proposed within probabilistic and exemplar views. See McGarty (1999) for a review.
2 For a discussion of different methodological paradigms to distinguish between analytical and non-analytical processes, see Cohen and Basu (1987) and Basu (1993).

Suggested readings

Alba, J.W. and Hutchinson, J.W. (1987) Dimensions of consumer expertise, *Journal of Consumer Research*, 13(4): 411–54. A review of research on consumer knowledge.
Alba, J.W. and Hutchinson, J.W. (1999) Applied cognition in consumer research, in F.T. Durso, R.S. Nickerson, R.W. Schaneveldt et al. (eds) *Handbook of Applied Cognition*. Chichester: Wiley. A review of cognitive processes involved in consumer judgement and decision making.
Alba, J.W. and Hutchinson, J.W. (2000) Knowledge calibration: what consumers know and what they think they know, *Journal of Consumer Research*, 27(2): 123–56. Another review of research on consumer knowledge.
John, D.R. (1999) Consumer socialization of children: a retrospective look at twenty-five years of research, *Journal of Consumer Research*, 26(3), 183–213. A review and future research directions in the area of children's cognitive development as consumers.
Kardes, F. (1994) Consumer judgement and decision processes, in R.S. Wyer Jr and T.K. Srull (eds) *Handbook of Social Cognition*, Vol. 2, *Applications*. Hillsdale, NJ: Erlbaum. A review of cognitive processes involved in consumer judgement and decision making.

Krishnan, H.S. and Chakravarti, D. (1999) Memory measures for pretesting advertisements: an integrative conceptual framework and a diagnostic temple, *Journal of Consumer Psychology*, 8(1): 1–37. A review of memory tests used for assessing advertising effectiveness.

Sit finis libri, non finis quaerendi . . .

Glossary

Accessibility: The activation potential of stored knowledge.

Action: What a person does either as a final performance or as a means to an end. Actions are bodily movements caused by mental states or events (for example beliefs, desires).

Action tendencies: A readiness to approach or avoid a goal object and usually experienced as an urge or impulse in response to a felt emotional reaction to a happening or to a change in progress towards achieving a goal. See also *coping responses*.

Affect: A broad term used to categorize such mental events or states as emotions, moods and (possibly) attitudes. Sometimes termed 'valenced feeling states'.

Affective commitment: A component of social identity reflecting the degree of emotional attachment or feeling of belongingness toward a focal group.

Amygdala: A region in the lower centre of the brain that acts as a kind of central processor and interacts with the prefrontal cortex (working memory and attention), hippocampus (long-term explicit memory) and sensory cortex (perception and short-term storage) to influence emotional processes.

Anticipated emotions: Positive and negative feelings expected if one were to envisage achieving and failing to achieve one's goal, respectively. Anticipated emotions influence desires and stimulate volitional processes. See *prefactuals*.

Appraisal theories: A class of theories maintaining that the critical determinants of any emotion are the judgements and interpretations a person makes after comparing an actual state to a desired state. See *emotion*.

Assimilation: The process by which a new concept is integrated into the schema.

Attention: The process by which an individual concentrates mental activity on a stimulus.

Attitude: A psychological tendency to respond evaluatively to persons, physical objects, ideas or actions in favourable or unfavourable ways.

Attitude accessibility: The strength of association between an attitude object and an evaluation in memory. It is measured how quickly attitude comes to mind and is an indication of attitude strength.

Attitude decay: The finding that initial persuasion (attitude change) dissipates over time, such that eventually an attitude returns to its original expression.

Attitude persistence: How long an attitude remains changed after persuasion.

Attitude resistance: The ability of an attitude to remain changed when presented with counter-persuasive information.

Attitude strength: An attitude dimension, theoretically unrelated to attitude extremity, that underlies the ability of an attitude to guide subsequent thought and behaviour.

Balance processes: Theories of attitude change based upon the notion that individuals prefer consistency (that is, balance) in their own attitudes, thoughts and behaviours (that is, intrapersonal balance) as well as their interpersonal relationships (that is, interpersonal balance). As a consequence, individuals are motivated to change their attitudes such that they are consistent with their own behaviour.

Belief: A thought about the property of an object (for example IBM computers are reliable) or the relationship (for example associational, causal, inferential) between two objects (for example regular use of Colgate toothpaste will lessen the buildup of plaque).

Belief elicitation: A procedure for identifying the set of modal salient beliefs of people that serve as inputs to or determinants of their attitudes.

Bookkeeping model: A schema change model which posits that each piece of new information leads to an incremental modification of the schema, and schema change occurs over time as perceivers are exposed to more incongruent information.

Categorization: The process of assigning an instance to a particular group or category.

Category-based induction: Generalization from one specific category (for example TVs) to a general category (for example all products).

Category exemplar: A specific instance or category member.

Category level: Categories can be represented at the basic (for example product type), subordinate (for example brand or specific products) and superordinate levels (for example product class). Whereas superordinate categories are generally described by abstract features, subordinate categories are associated with more specific features.

Category prototype: A summary representation or an abstraction that best represents a category.

Central route: Attitude change that is the result of elaboration.

Circumplex model: A categorization of emotions based on the blending of combinations of emotions formed by crossing two factors: pleasure–displeasure and arousal–sleepiness (or alternatively, high positive affect–low positive affect and high negative affect–low negative affect). For example, fear can be thought of as a combination of high arousal and displeasure, depression as a combination of displeasure and low arousal (sleepiness), and joy as a combination of high arousal and pleasure.

Cognitive dissonance: Theory of attitude change based upon the notion that attitudes are changed in order to reduce internal feelings of discomfort that arise in response to becoming aware of inconsistencies between our attitudes and behaviour.

Cognitive identification: A component of social identity reflecting the extent of awareness that one is a member of a focal group. Also known as self-categorization.

Cognitive responses: The idiosyncratic thoughts and reactions that an individual has in response to persuasive information.

Cognitive response approach: Theory of attitude change based upon the notion that individuals are persuaded by their own idiosyncratic thoughts and reactions to persuasive information.

Consumer behaviour: The psychological and social processes people undergo in the acquisition, use, and disposal of products, services, ideas and practices.

Coping responses: Actions or mental activities taken to restore equilibrium perturbed by the experience of an emotion. Problem-focused coping attempts to alleviate the sources of distress. Emotion-focused coping tries to change the meaning of the source of distress or avoid thinking about a problem. See also *action tendencies*.

Conversion model: A schema change model which posits that schemas change when exposed to extremely atypical instances.

Desire: A motivational state directed at either a goal or an act and existing in two forms: appetitive (for example a craving, longing, yearning, urge, hunger, appetite) and volitive (for example a want, wish). Desires are thought to transform reasons for acting (for example attitudes, beliefs, subjective norms) into intentions or decisions to act. See *second-order desire*.

Dual route models: Theories that allow for two distinct psychological processes. Most typically, one of the processes is thoughtful in nature, while the other process is relatively non-thoughtful.

Elaboration: The psychological process of attitude change in which individuals thoughtfully consider the information presented, generate thoughts and feelings in response to that information, and change their attitude as a function of these cognitive responses. See *thoughtful attitude change*.

Emotion: A mental state of readiness that arises from cognitive appraisals of events or thoughts, has a phenomenological tone, is accompanied by physiological processes, is often expressed physically, and may result in specific actions to affirm or cope with the emotion.

Encoding specificity principle: Retrieval cues improve memory performance only when they are specifically encoded with the target information.

Epiphenomenalism: Philosophical doctrine maintaining that mental events (for example beliefs, attitudes) are caused by common physical events in the brain but do not cause each other or actions.

Evaluation: A judgement of the value of something expressed by such bipolar adjectives as good–bad, favourable–unfavourable, punishing–rewarding, wise–foolish and useful–useless.

Evaluative (collective) self-esteem: A component of social identity reflecting the extent that one feels one is an important, valued member of a focal group.

Expectancy-value model: Representation of a person's attitude as the sum of the products of beliefs about the attributes of an object (or the consequences of an act) times the evaluations of the attributes (or consequences of an act). In some versions of the model, evaluations are replaced by importances, satisfaction or affective responses. Although generally conceived as a unidimensional representation of an attitude, the expectancy-value model has been used to represent multidimensional responses to the same target object or act or to a goal (for example toward trying and succeeding, trying and failing, and striving, per se).

Family resemblance: A determinant of typicality in categories and defined as an exemplar's similarity to the central tendency of its category.

Frequency of instantiation: A determinant of typicality and refers to perceived estimates of how often an instance is encountered as a member of the category.

Goal: Mental representation of either an object that a person wants to acquire, an outcome one desires to produce, or an action one wishes to perform.

Goal efficacy: The perceived likelihood of goal achievement, given that one decides to try to achieve a goal. Similar to *outcome expectancies*.

Goal intention: A decision to pursue a goal. Goal intentions are functions of the interaction between goal desires and second-order desires.

Graded structure: Category members and non-members varying in their similarity to the category.

Halo effect: The finding that attitudes influence beliefs (or alternatively expectancy-value reactions) in contradistinction to the opposite sequence, which is more commonly presumed.

Implementation intention: A decision to pursue a goal-directed behaviour and is expressed conditionally on the occurrence of future contingencies: 'I intend to do X when situation Y is encountered'. Implementation intentions are thought to accompany planning as to when, where, how, and how long one is to act.

Intention: A decision to pursue a goal or perform an action. Often intentions are taken to include a certain degree of motivation or commitment to act. See *goal intention* and *implementation intention*.

Long-term memory: The system for permanently storing information for later use.

Means-end chain theory: The organization of consumer knowledge in a hierarchy with concrete thoughts linked to more abstract thoughts in a sequence progressing from *means* to *ends*. One usage of the theory focuses upon this sequence: beliefs about physical product attributes→psychosocial consequences→values. The hierarchy of 'thoughts' can also consist of goals, motives or values.

Mere exposure effect: Attitude change occurring as a function of repeated exposure to an object that is simple, previously unknown, and contains little or no semantic content.

Modal salient beliefs: The set of attitude-forming beliefs that are notable and relevant in a given population of individuals.

MODE model: 'Motivation and opportunity as determinants of how attitudes influence behaviour'. Fazio's (1986, 1990) hypothesis that behaviour can be spontaneously produced when an attitude is activated. An attitude can be automatically activated from memory by observation of either an attitude object or cues associated with the object, depending on the extent of attitude accessibility.

Model of goal-directed behaviour: Comprehensive theory of action that maintains that behaviour is influenced by intentions and recency and frequency of past performance of the behaviour; intentions are determined by desires, frequency of past performance of the behaviour, and perceived behavioural control; and desires are functions of attitude, positive anticipated emotions, negative anticipated emotions, subjective norms and perceived behavioural control.

Mood: A subjective positive or negative feeling state that is longer lasting than an emotion and unlike an emotion is generally non-intentional (that is, it has no object or referent) and is more global or diffused. Moods are not as directly coupled with action tendencies and action as are emotions.

Motivation to comply: Felt need to acquiesce to the expectations of specific significant others.

Multiple roles: Variables can influence persuasion by either (a) serving as a peripheral cue, (b) influencing the extent of elaboration, (c) serving as an argument, or (d) influencing the nature of the thoughts. The overall elaboration likelihood influences by which role a variable guides persuasion.

Need for cognition: Need for cognition measures an individual's intrinsic enjoyment of and motivation to thoughtfully consider information. As such, individuals high in need for cognition enjoy elaborating, and demonstrate a proclivity to elaborate persuasive information, even when situational influences do not prompt such consideration. In contrast, individuals low in need for cognition do not enjoy elaborating, and tend to rely upon non-thoughtful persuasion processes.

Non-thoughtful attitude change: The psychological process of attitude change in which individuals rely upon (a) less effortful scrutiny of the issue-relevant information, (b) inference processes, and/or (c) associative processes rather than elaboration.

Normative beliefs: Felt expectations from specific others whose opinions are valued to the effect that one should or should not act.

Outcome expectancies: Perceived likelihood that one will achieve an outcome. Similar to goal efficacy.

Perceived behavioural control: A person's belief as to the ease or difficulty of performing a prospective behaviour. Perceived behavioural control influences intentions and, as a proxy for actual control, influences behaviour. It is modelled as the sums of products of beliefs that one has access to factors needed to perform a behaviour, and the perceived power of the factors contributing to the behaviour.

Perception: A mental process that uses previous knowledge to compile and interpret the stimuli that are registered by our senses.

Peripheral route: Attitude change that is the result of non-thoughtful inferences and associations.

Persuasion: The extent to which an attitude changes.

Preattentive processing: The non-conscious processing of stimuli in peripheral vision.

Prefactuals: Forward-looking counterfactual thinking of the sort embodied in anticipated happenings and their implications for oneself. See *anticipated emotions.*

Priming: Activation of a stored knowledge unit, which increases its accessibility and consequently its effect on a subsequent judgement, given that it is relevant and other concepts are not chronically accessible.

Proactive interference: Memory performance can be reduced as a function of learning additional related information before the target is encountered.

Prospective memory: Remembering to perform an action at a future point in time.

Retroactive interference: Memory performance can be reduced as a function of learning additional related information after the target is encountered.

Satisfaction: Subjective feeling state used by researchers to measure reactions of consumers to product or service performance.

Schemas: Cognitive structures that represent organized knowledge about different categories such as self, other people, events and objects.

Script: Organized knowledge structure about sequences of events in a period of time.

Second-order desire: Self-evaluative or moral standards concerning who a person is and desires to be. Second-order desires moderate the effects of goal desires on goal intentions and behavioural desires on implementation desires. See *desire.*

Self-categorization: A component of social identity reflecting the extent of awareness that one is a member of a focal group. Also known as cognitive identification.

Self-efficacy: The confidence one has that one can perform a particular behaviour.

Self-perception: Theory of attitude change based upon the notion that individuals infer their attitudes from their own behaviour.

Semantic differential: Bipolar scales used to measure attitudes or evaluations and expressed typically on 5-point or 7-point items anchored by such adjectives as good–bad, useful–useless and wise–foolish.

Sensory memory: Temporary storage of the information received from senses.

Short-term memory: Portion of memory, with limited capacity, for interpreting information from existing knowledge. For example, you are using short-term memory to comprehend this sentence.

Simultaneity: A claim that attitudes and expectancy-value reactions are related reciprocally, as opposed to the more commonly presumed sequence of expectancy-value reactions→attitudes.

Social identity: Representation of a person's identity as a consequence of group membership. Three components are proposed: self-categorization, affective commitment and evaluative or collective self-esteem.

Somatic marker hypothesis: The biasing of the evaluation of goal objects and other antecedents to decision making by unconscious preferences stored as nondeclarative dispositional knowledge.

Subjective norm: Perceived social pressure to perform or not perform an act as felt through the expectations of persons whose opinions one values. Subjective normative pressure is believed to be based on the need for approval and is sometimes termed, compliance. Subjective norms influence intentions and are modelled as functions of the sums of products of normative beliefs and motivation to comply with the expectations of significant others.

Subtyping: The process by which inconsistent category members are set apart and considered unrepresentative of the category.

Theory of planned behaviour: A model of action that asserts that behaviour is a direct function of intentions to act and perceived behavioural control; while intentions to act are functions of attitudes toward the act, felt subjective norms to act, and perceived behavioural control.

Theory of reasoned action: A model of action that claims that behaviour is a direct function of intentions to act and intentions to act are functions, in turn, of attitudes toward the act and felt subjective norms to act.

Theory of self-regulation: An expansion of the theory of trying that posits the following sequence of effects: goal desire→goal intention→trying→instrumental actions →goal attainment/failure. In addition, goal desires are hypothesized to transform the effects of five reasons for choosing a goal: goal efficacy, attitude toward success, attitude toward failure, attitude toward the process or means of goal striving and subjective norms. Also expectations of success and failure might moderate the effects of attitudes toward success and failure, respectively, on goal desires.

Theory of trying: A model of action that maintains that behaviour is a direct function of trying to act, trying to act is a function of intentions to act, and intentions to act are functions of attitudes toward success, attitudes toward failure, attitudes toward the process of goal pursuit and subjective norms. In some versions of the theory, attitudes towards success and failure interact with expectations of success and failure, respectively, to influence intentions.

Thoughtful attitude change: Elaboration.

Trustworthiness: The extent to which a source of information can be trusted to provide accurate information.

Trying: The mental and physical activities needed to initiate and regulate instrumental acts. Under the narrow view of trying, it refers to volition, planning, monitoring of progress towards a goal, guidance and control activities, maintenance of commitment, and willpower. Under the broad view, intention and/or instrumental acts targeted at a goal are added to the criteria under the narrow view. Trying serves to transform the decision or intention to act into observed bodily movements directed at goal attainment. See *volition*.

Values: Criteria people use to select and justify goals and actions. Often categorized into instrumental and terminal varieties.

Volition: The mental faculty of willing or trying to act. Volition is thought to be the mental event that produces bodily movements (that is, action or behaviour). See *trying*.

References

Aaker, D.A. and Keller, K.L. (1990) Consumer evaluations of brand extensions, *Journal of Marketing*, 54: 27–41.

Aaker, D.A., Stayman, D.M. and Hagerty, M.R. (1986) Warmth in advertising: measurement, impact and sequence effects, *Journal of Consumer Research*, 12: 365–81.

Aaker, D.A., Stayman, D.M. and Vezina, R. (1988) Identifying feelings elicited by advertising, *Psychology and Marketing*, 5: 1–16.

Aaker, J.L. (1999) The malleable self: the role of self-expression in persuasion, *Journal of Marketing Research*, 36: 45–57.

Aaker, J.L. (2000) Accessibility or diagnosticity? Disentangling the influence of culture on persuasion processes and attitudes, *Journal of Consumer Research*, 26: 340–57.

Aaker, J.L. and Lee, A.Y. (2001) 'I' seek pleasures and 'we' avoid pains: the role of self regulatory goals in information processing and persuasion, *Journal of Consumer Research*, 28(1): 33–49.

Aarts, H. and Dijksterhuis, A. (2000) Habit as knowledge structure: automaticity in goal-directed behavior, *Journal of Personality and Social Psychology*, 78: 53–63.

Abelson, R.P., Aronson, E., McGuire, W.J. et al. (1968) *Theories of Cognitive Consistency: A Sourcebook*. Chicago: Rand McNally.

Ahluwalia, R. and Gürhan-Canli, Z. (2000) The effects of extensions on the family brand name: an accessibility-diagnosticity perspective, *Journal of Consumer Research*, 27: 371–81.

Ahluwalia, R., Burnkrant, R. and Unnava, R. (2000) Consumer responses to negative publicity: the moderating role of commitment, *Journal of Marketing Research*, 37: 203–14.

Ajzen, I. (1985) From intentions to actions: a theory of planned behavior, in J. Kuhl and J. Beckmann (eds) *Action Control: From Cognition to Behavior*. New York: Springer-Verlag.

Ajzen, I. (1991) The theory of planned behavior, *Organizational Behavior and Human Decision Processes*, 50: 179–211.

Ajzen, I. and Driver, B.E. (1991) Prediction of leisure participation from behavioural, normative, and control beliefs: an application of the theory of planned behavior, *Leisure Studies*, 13: 185–204.

Ajzen, I. and Driver, B.L. (1992) Application of the theory of planned behavior to leisure choice, *Journal of Leisure Research*, 24: 207–24.

Ajzen, I. and Fishbein, M. (1977) Attitude–behavior relations: a theoretical analysis and review of empirical research, *Psychological Bulletin*, 84: 888–918.

Ajzen, I. and Fishbein, M. (1980) *Understanding Attitudes and Predicting Social Behavior*. Englewood Cliffs, NJ: Prentice-Hall.

Ajzen, I. and Madden, T.J. (1986) Predictions of goal-directed behavior: attitudes, intentions, and perceived behavioral control, *Journal of Experimental Social Psychology*, 22: 453–74.

Alba, J.W. and Hutchinson, J.W. (1987) Dimensions of consumer expertise, *Journal of Consumer Research*, 13: 411–53.

Alba, J.W., Broniarczk, S.M., Shimp, T.A. and Urbany, J.E. (1994) The influence of prior beliefs, frequency cues, and magnitude cues on consumers' perceptions of comparative price data, *Journal of Consumer Research*, 21: 219–35.

Alba, J.W., Mela, C.F., Shimp, T.A. and Urbany, J.E. (1999) The effect of discount frequency and depth on consumer price judgements, *Journal of Consumer Research*, 26: 99–114.

Allen, C.T. and Janiszewski, C.A. (1989) Assessing the role of contingency awareness in attitudinal conditioning with implications for advertising research, *Journal of Marketing Research*, 26: 30–43.

Allen, C., Machleit, K. and Kleine, S.S. (1992) A comparison of attitudes and emotions as predictors of behavior at diverse levels of behavioral experience, *Journal of Consumer Research*, 18: 493–504.

Allen, M. (1983) Models of hemispheric specialization, *Psychological Bulletin*, 93: 73–104.

Allport, G.W. (1935) Attitudes, in C.A. Murchinson (ed.) *A Handbook of Social Psychology*. Worcester, MA: Clark University Press.

Anderson, J.R. (1980) *Cognitive Psychology and its Implications*. San Francisco, CA: Freeman.

Anderson, J.R. (1983) *The Architecture of Cognition*. Cambridge, MA: Harvard University Press.

Anderson, N.H. (1981) *Foundations of Information Integration Theory*. San Diego, CA: Academic Press.

Armitage, C.J. and Conner, M. (1999) Distinguishing perceptions of control from self-efficacy: predicting consumption of a low-fat diet using the theory of planned behavior, *Journal of Applied Social Psychology*, 29: 72–90.

Armitage, C.J. and Conner, M. (2001) Efficacy of the theory of planned behaviour: a meta-analytic review, *British Journal of Social Psychology*, 40: 471–99.

Atkinson, R.C. and Shiffrin, R.M. (1968) Human memory: a proposed system and its control processes, in K.W. Spence and J.T. Spence (eds) *The Psychology of Learning and Motivation: Advances in Research and Theory*. New York: Academic Press.

Audenaert, A. and Steenkamp, J-B.E.M. (1997) Means-end chain theory and laddering in agricultural marketing research, in B. Wierenga, A. van Tilburg, K. Grunert, J-B.E.M. Steenkamp and M. Wedel (eds) *Agricultural Marketing and Consumer Behaviour in a Changing World*. Amsterdam: Kluwer.

Austin, J.T. and Vancouver, J.B. (1996) Goal constructs in psychology: structure, process, and content, *Psychological Bulletin*, 120: 338–75.

Bagozzi, R.P. (1978) The construct validity of the affective, behavioural, and cognitive components of attitude by analysis of covariance structures, *Multivariate Behavioral Research*, 13: 9–31.

Bagozzi, R.P. (1980) *Causal Models in Marketing*. New York: Wiley.

Bagozzi, R.P. (1981a) An examination of the validity of two models of attitude, *Multivariate Behavioral Research*, 16: 323–59.

Bagozzi, R.P. (1981b) Attitudes, intentions, and behavior: a test of some key hypotheses, *Journal of Personality and Social Psychology*, 41: 607–27.

Bagozzi, R.P. (1982) A field investigation of causal relations among cognitions, affect, intentions, and behavior, *Journal of Marketing Research*, 19: 562–84.

Bagozzi, R.P. (1984) Expectancy-value attitude models: an analysis of critical measurement issues, *International Journal of Research in Marketing*, 1: 295–310.

Bagozzi, R.P. (1985) Expectancy-value attitude models: an analysis of critical theoretical issues, *International Journal of Research in Marketing*, 2: 43–60.

Bagozzi, R.P. (1986) Attitude formation under the theory of reasoned action and a purposeful behaviour reformulation, *British Journal of Social Psychology*, 25: 95–107.

Bagozzi, R.P. (1989) An investigation of the role of affective and moral evaluations in the purposive behaviour model of attitude, *British Journal of Social Psychology*, 28: 97–113.

Bagozzi, R.P. (1991a) Further thoughts on the validity of measures of elation, gladness, and joy, *Journal of Personality and Social Psychology*, 61: 98–104.

Bagozzi, R.P. (1991b) The role of psychophysiology in consumer research, in T.S. Robertson and H.H. Kassarjian (eds) *Handbook of Consumer Behavior*. Englewood Cliffs, NJ: Prentice-Hall.

Bagozzi, R.P. (1992) The self-regulation of attitudes, intentions, and behavior, *Social Psychology Quarterly*, 55: 178–204.

Bagozzi, R.P. (1993) An examination of the psychometric properties of measures of negative affect in the PANAS-X scales, *Journal of Personality and Social Psychology*, 65: 836–51.

Bagozzi, R.P. (1994a) *Principles of Marketing Research*. Oxford: Blackwell.

Bagozzi, R.P. (1994b) The effects of arousal on the organization of positive and negative affect and cognitions: application to attitude theory, *Structural Equation Modeling*, 1: 222–52.

Bagozzi, R.P. (1994c) *Principles of Marketing Research*. Oxford: Blackwell.

Bagozzi, R.P. (1996) The role of arousal in the creation and control of the halo effect in attitude models, *Psychology and Marketing*, 13: 235–64.

Bagozzi, R.P. (1999) Happiness, in D. Levinson, J. Ponzetti and P. Jorgenson (eds) *Encyclopedia of Human Emotions*. New York: Macmillan.

Bagozzi, R.P. (2000a) On the concept of intentional social action in consumer behavior, *Journal of Consumer Research*, 27: 388–96.

Bagozzi, R.P. (2000b) The poverty of economic explanations of consumption and an action theory alternative, *Managerial and Decision Economics*, 21: 95–109.

Bagozzi, R.P. and Burnkrant, R.E. (1979) Attitude organization and the attitude-behavior relationship, *Journal of Personality and Social Psychology*, 37: 913–29.

Bagozzi, R.P. and Burnkrant, R.E. (1985) Attitude organization and the attitude–behavior relation: a reply to Dillon and Kumar, *Journal of Personality and Social Psychology*, 49: 47–57.

Bagozzi, R.P. and Dabholkar, P.A. (2000) Discursive psychology: an alternative conceptual foundation to means-end chain theory, *Psychology and Marketing*, 17: 535–86.

Bagozzi, R.P. and Dholakia, U. (1999) Goal-setting and goal-striving in consumer behavior, *Journal of Marketing*, 63: 19–32.

Bagozzi, R.P. and Dholakia, U.M. (2002) Intentional social action in virtual communities, *Journal of Interactive Marketing*, 16: 2–21.

Bagozzi, R.P. and Edwards, E.A. (1998) Goal setting and goal pursuit in the regulation of body weight, *Psychology and Health*, 13: 593–621.

Bagozzi, R.P. and Edwards, E.A. (2000) Goal-striving and the implementation of goal intentions in the regulation of body weight, *Psychology and Health*, 15: 255–70.

Bagozzi, R.P. and Kimmel, S.K. (1995) A comparison of leading theories for the prediction of goal-directed behaviours, *British Journal of Social Psychology*, 34: 437–61.

Bagozzi, R.P. and Lee, K-H. (2001) Intentional social action and the reasons why we do things with others. Unpublished working paper, Rice University.

Bagozzi, R.P. and Lee, K-H. (2002) Multiple routes for social influence: the role of compliance, internalization, and social identity, *Social Psychology Quarterly*.

Bagozzi, R.P. and Moore, D.J. (1994) Public service advertisements: emotion and empathy guide prosocial behavior, *Journal of Marketing*, 58: 56–70.

Bagozzi, R.P. and Warshaw, P.R. (1990) Trying to consume, *Journal of Consumer Research*, 17: 127–40.

Bagozzi, R.P. and Warshaw, P.R. (1992) An examination of the etiology of the attitude–behavior relation for goal-directed behaviors, *Multivariate Behavioral Research*, 27: 601–34.

Bagozzi, R.P. and Yi, Y. (1989) The degree of intention formation as a moderator of the attitude–behavior relationship, *Social Psychology Quarterly*, 52: 266–79.

Bagozzi, R.P., Baumgartner, J. and Yi, Y. (1989) An investigation into the role of intentions as mediators of the attitude–behavior relationship, *Journal of Economic Psychology*, 10: 35–62.

Bagozzi, R.P., Yi, Y. and Baumgartner, J. (1990) The level of effort required for behaviour as a moderator of the attitude–behaviour relation, *European Journal of Social Psychology*, 20: 45–59.

Bagozzi, R.P., Baumgartner, H. and Yi, Y. (1992a) Appraisal processes in the enactment of intentions to use coupons, *Psychology & Marketing*, 9: 469–86.

Bagozzi, R.P., Baumgartner, H. and Yi, Y. (1992b) State- vs. action-orientation and the theory of reasoned action: an application to coupon usage, *Journal of Consumer Research*, 18: 505–18.

Bagozzi, R.P., Davis, F.D. and Warshaw, P.R. (1992c) Development and test of a theory of technological learning and usage, *Human Relations*, 45: 659–86.

Bagozzi, R.P., Baumgartner, H. and Pieters, R. (1998) Goal-directed emotions, *Cognition and Emotion*, 12: 1–16.

Bagozzi, R.P., Gopinath, M. and Nyer, P.U. (1999a) *Journal of the Academy of Marketing Science*, 27: 184–206.

Bagozzi, R.P., Wong, N. and Yi, Y. (1999b) The role of culture and gender in the relationship between positive and negative affect, *Cognition and Emotion*, 13: 641–72.

Bagozzi, R.P., Bergami, M. and Leone, L. (2001a) Hierarchical representation of motives in goal-setting. Paper under review.

Bagozzi, R.P., Lee, K-H. and Van Loo, M.F. (2001b) Decisions to donate bone marrow: the role of attitudes and subjective norms across cultures, *Psychology and Health*, 16: 29–56.

Bagozzi, R.P., Moore, D.J. and Leone, L. (2001c) Self-control and the regulation of dieting: the role of prefactual attitudes, subjective norms, and resistance to temptation. Paper under review.

Baker, S.M. and Petty, R.E. (1994) Majority and minority influence: source-position imbalance as a determinant of message scrutiny, *Journal of Personality and Social Psychology*, 67: 5–19.

Bandura, A. (1994) *Self-efficacy: The Exercise of Control*. New York: Freeman.

Bargh, J.A. and Barndollar, K. (1996) Automaticity in action: the unconscious as repository of chronic goals and motives, in P.M. Gollwitzer and J.A. Bargh (eds) *The Psychology of Action: Linking Cognition and Motivation to Behavior*. New York: Guilford.

Bargh, J.A., Chaiken, S., Govender, R. and Pratto, F. (1992) The generality of the automatic attitude activation effect, *Journal of Personality and Social Psychology*, 62: 893–912.

Barone, M.J., Miniard, P.W. and Romeo, J.B. (2000) The influence of positive mood on brand extension evaluations, *Journal of Consumer Research*, 26: 386–400.

Barrett, L.F. and Russell, J.A. (1998) Independence and bipolarity in the structure of current affect, *Journal of Personality and Social Psychology*, 74: 967–84.

Barsalou, L.W. (1985) Ideals, central tendency, and frequency of instantiation as determinants of graded structure in categories, *Journal of Experimental Psychology: Learning, Memory, and Cognition*, 11: 629–54.

Barsalou, L.W. (1991) Deriving categories to achieve goals, in G.H. Bower (ed.) *The Psychology of Learning and Motivation*, Vol. 27. New York: Academic Press.

Bartlett, J.C. and Santrock, J.W. (1979) Affect-dependent episodic memory in young children, *Child Development*, 50: 513–18.

Bartlett, J.C., Burleson, G. and Santrock, J.W. (1982) Emotional mood and memory in young children, *Journal of Experimental Child Psychology*, 34: 59–76.

Bassili, J.N. (1996) Meta-judgemental versus operative indexes of psychological attributes: the case of measures of attitude strength, *Journal of Personality and Social Psychology*, 71: 637–53.

Basu, K. (1993) Consumers' categorization processes: an examination with two alternative methodological paradigms, *Journal of Consumer Psychology*, 2: 97–121.

Batra, R. and Holbrook, M.B. (1990) Developing a typology of affective responses to advertising, *Psychology and Marketing*, 7: 11–25.

Batra, R. and Ray, M.L. (1986) Affective responses mediating acceptance of advertising, *Journal of Consumer Research*, 13: 234–49.

Batra, R. and Stayman, D.M. (1990) The role of mood in advertising effectiveness, *Journal of Consumer Research*, 17: 203–14.

Batra, R. and Stephens, D. (1994) Attitudinal effects of ad-evoked moods and emotions: the moderating role of motivation, *Psychology and Marketing*, 11: 199–215.

Bechara, A., Damasio, H., Tranel, D. and Damasio, A.R. (1997) Deciding advantageously before knowing the advantageous strategy, *Science*, 275: 1293–5.

Beck, L. and Ajzen, I. (1991) Predicting dishonest actions using the theory of planned behavior, *Journal of Research in Personality*, 25: 285–301.

Bem, D.J. (1972) Self-perception theory, in L. Berkowitz (ed.) *Advances in Experimental Social Psychology*, Vol. 6. New York: Academic Press.

Bentler, P.M. and Speckart, G. (1979) Models of attitude–behavior relations, *Psychological Review*, 86: 452–64.

Bentler, P.M. and Speckart, G. (1981) Attitudes cause behaviors: a structural equation analysis, *Journal of Personality and Social Psychology*, 40: 226–38.

Berg, K.E. (1966) Ethnic attitudes and agreement with a Negro person, *Journal of Personality and Social Psychology*, 4: 215–20.

Bergami, M. and Bagozzi, R.P. (2000) Self-categorisation, affective commitment, and group self-esteem as distinct aspects of social identity in the organisation, *British Journal of Social Psychology*, 39: 555–77.

Bettman, J.R., Capon, N. and Lutz, R.J. (1975) Information processing in attitude formation and change, *Communication Research*, 2: 267–78.

Bettman, J.R., Luce, M.R. and Payne, J.W. (1998) Constructive consumer processes, *Journal of Consumer Research*, 25: 187–217.

Bishop, J. (1989) *Natural Agency: An Essay on the Causal Theory of Action*. Cambridge: Cambridge University Press.

Bitner, M.J. (1990) Evaluating service encounters: the effects of physical surroundings and employee responses, *Journal of Marketing*, 54: 69–82.

Blackburn, S. (1994) *The Oxford Dictionary of Philosophy*. Oxford: Oxford University Press.

Blascovitch, J., Ernst, J.M., Tomaka, J. et al. (1993) Attitude accessibility as a moderator of autonomic reactivity during decision making, *Journal of Personality and Social Psychology*, 64: 165–76.

Bless, H., Bohner, G.L., Schwarz, G.N. and Strack, F. (1990) Mood and persuasion: a cognitive response analysis, *Personality and Social Psychology Bulletin*, 16(2): 331–45.

Bless, H., Clore, G.L., Schwarz, N. et al. (1996) Mood and the use of scripts: does a happy mood really lead to mindlessness?, *Journal of Personality and Social Psychology*, 71(4): 665–79.

Block, L.G. and Morwitz, V.G. (1999) Shopping lists as an external memory aid for grocery shopping: influences on list writing and list fulfillment, *Journal of Consumer Psychology*, 8: 343–75.

Bodenhausen, G.V. (1988) Stereotypic biases in social decision making and memory: testing process models of stereotype use, *Journal of Personality and Social Psychology*, 55: 726–37.

Bohner, G., Crow, K., Erb, H-P. and Schwarz, N. (1992) Affect and persuasion: mood effects on the processing of message content and context cues and on subsequent behaviour, *European Journal of Social Psychology*, 22: 511–30.

Boninger, D.S., Gleicher, F. and Strathman, A. (1994a) Counterfactual thinking: from what might have been to what may be, *Journal of Personality and Social Psychology*, 67: 297–307.

Boninger, D.S., Gleicher, F., Hetts, J., Armor, D. and Moore, E. (1994b) The influence of counterfactual thinking on intentions and behavior. Unpublished raw data, reported in F. Gleicher, D.S. Boninger, A. Strathman et al. (1995).

Bower, G.H. (1981) Mood and memory, *American Psychologist*, 36(2): 129–48.

Bower, G.H. and Cohen, P.R. (1982) Emotional influences in memory and thinking: data and theory, in M.S. Clark and S.T. Fiske (eds) *Affect and Cognition*. Hillsdale, NJ: Erlbaum.

Bower, G.H. and Mayer, J.D. (1985) Failure to replicate mood-dependent retrieval, *Bulletin of the Psychonomic Society*, 23: 39–42.

Bower, G.H., Montiero, K.P. and Gilligan, S.G. (1978) Emotional mood as a context for learning and recall, *Journal of Verbal Learning and Verbal Behavior*, 17: 573–85.

Bower, G.H., Gilligan, S.G. and Montiero, K.P. (1981) Selectivity of learning caused by affective states, *Journal of Experimental Psychology: General*, 110(4): 451–73.

Bozzolo, A.M. and Brock, T.C. (1992) Unavailability effects on message processing: a theoretical analysis and an empirical test, *Basic and Applied Social Psychology*, 13: 93–101.

Bradburn, N.M. (1969) *The Structure of Psychological Well-Being*. Chicago: Aldine.

Bratman, M.E. (1987) *Intentions, Plans, and Practical Reason*. Cambridge, MA: Harvard University Press.

Braun, K.A. (1999) Postexperience advertising effects on consumer memory, *Journal of Consumer Research*, 25: 319–34.

Bray, D.W. (1950) The prediction of behaviour from two attitude scales, *Journal of Abnormal and Social Psychology*, 45: 64–84.

Breckler, S.J. (1984) Empirical validation of affect, behavior, and cognition as distinct components of attitude, *Journal of Personality and Social Psychology*, 47: 1191–205.

Breckler, S.J. and Wiggins, E.C. (1989) Affect versus evaluation in the structure of attitudes, *Journal of Experimental Social Psychology*, 25: 253–71.

Brewer, M.B. (1988) A dual process model of impression formation, in T.K. Srull and R.S. Wyer (eds) *Advances in Social Cognition*, Vol. 1. Hillsdale, NJ: Lawrence Erlbaum Associates.

Broniarczyk, S.M. and Alba, J.W. (1994a) The importance of the brand in brand extension, *Journal of Marketing Research*, 31: 214–28.

Broniarczyk, S.M. and Alba, J.W. (1994b) The role of consumers' intuitions in inference making, *Journal of Consumer Research*, 21: 393–407.

Broniarczyk, S.M., Hoyer, W.D. and McAlister, L. (1998) Consumers' perceptions of the assortment offered in a grocery category: the impact of item reduction, *Journal of Marketing Research*, 35: 166–76.

Brown, S.P. and Stayman, D.M. (1992) Antecedents and consequences of attitude toward the ad: a meta-analysis, *Journal of Consumer Research*, 19: 34–51.

Brown, T.J. and Dacin, P.A. (1997) The company and the product: corporate associations and consumer product responses, *Journal of Marketing*, 61: 68–84.

Brown, T.J. and Rothschild, M.L. (1993) Reassessing the impact of television advertising clutter, *Journal of Consumer Research*, 20: 138–46.

Brucks, M. (1985) The effects of product class knowledge on information search behavior, *Journal of Consumer Research*, 12: 1–16.

Budd, R.J. (1986) Predicting cigarette use: the need to incorporate measures of salience in the theory of reasoned action, *Journal of Applied Social Psychology*, 16: 663–85.

Burke, M.C. and Edell, J.A. (1989) The impact of feelings on ad-based affect and cognition, *Journal of Marketing Research*, 26: 69–83.

Burke, R.R. and Srull, T.K. (1988) Competitive interference and consumer memory for advertising, *Journal of Consumer Research*, 15: 55–68.

Burnkrant, R.E. and Howard, D.J. (1984) Effects of the use of introductory rhetorical questions versus statements on information processing, *Journal of Personality and Social Psychology*, 47: 1218–30.

Burnkrant, R.E. and Unnava, R. (1989) Self-referencing: a strategy increasing processing of message content, *Personality and Social Psychology Bulletin*, 15: 628–38.

Cacioppo, J.T. and Petty, R.E. (1979) Attitudes and cognitive response: an electrophysiological approach, *Journal of Personality and Social Psychology*, 37: 2181–99.

Cacioppo, J.T. and Petty, R.E. (1981) Effects of extent of thought on the pleasantness ratings of P-O-X triads: evidence for three judgemental tendencies in evaluating social situation, *Journal of Personality and Social Psychology*, 40: 1000–9.

Cacioppo, J.T. and Petty, R.E. (1982) The need for cognition, *Journal of Personality and Social Psychology*, 42: 116–31.

Cacioppo, J.T. and Petty, R.E. (1989) Effects of message repetition on argument processing, recall, and persuasion, *Basic and Applied Social Psychology*, 10: 3–12.

Cacioppo, J.T., Harkins, S.G. and Petty, R.E. (1981) The nature of attitudes and cognitive responses and their relationships to behavior, in R.E. Petty, T.M. Ostrom and T.C. Brock (eds) *Cognitive Responses in Persuasion*. Mahwah, NJ: Erlbaum.

Cacioppo, J.T., Petty, R.E. and Morris, K. (1983) Effects of need for cognition on message evaluation, recall, and persuasion, *Journal of Personality and Social Psychology*, 45: 805–18.

Cacioppo, J.T., Petty, R.E. and Kao, C. (1984a) The efficient assessment of need for cognition, *Journal of Personality Assessment*, 48: 306–7.

Cacioppo, J.T., Petty, R.E. and Marshall-Goodell, B. (1984b) Electromyographic specificity during simple physical and attitudinal tasks: location and topographical features of integrated EMG responses, *Biological Psychology*, 18: 85–121.

Cacioppo, J.T., Petty, R.E. and Morris, K. (1985) Semantic, evaluative, and self-referent processing: memory, cognitive effort, and somatovisceral activity, *Psychophysiology*, 22: 371–84.

Cacioppo, J.T., Petty, R.E., Kao, C. and Rodriguez, R. (1986a) Central and peripheral routes to persuasion: an individual difference perspective, *Journal of Personality and Social Psychology*, 51: 1032–43.

Cacioppo, J.R., Petty, R.E., Losch, M.L. and Kim, H.S. (1986b) Electromyographic activity over facial muscle regions can differentiate the valence and intensity of affective reactions, *Journal of Personality and Social Psychology*, 50: 260–8.

Cacioppo, J.T., Berntson, G.G. and Klein, D.J. (1992a) What is an emotion? The role of somatovisceral afference, with special emphasis on somatovisceral 'illusions', *Review of Personality and Social Psychology*, 14: 63–98.

Cacioppo, J.T., Marshall-Goodell, B.S., Tassinary, L.G. and Petty, R.E. (1992b) Rudimentary determinants of attitudes: classical conditioning is more effective when prior knowledge about the attitude stimulus is low than high, *Journal of Experimental Social Psychology*, 28: 207–33.

Cacioppo, J.T., Priester, J.R. and Berntson, G. (1993) Rudimentary determinants of Attitudes II: arm flexion and extension have differential effects on attitudes, *Journal of Personality and Social Psychology*, 65: 5–17.

Cacioppo, J.T., Petty, R.E., Feinstein, J. and Jarvis, W.B.G. (1996) Dispositional differences in cognitive motivation: the life and times of individuals varying in need for cognition, *Psychological Bulletin*, 119: 197–253.

Calder, B.J. and Ross, M. (1973) *Attitudes and Behavior*. Morristown, NJ: General Learning Press.

Campbell, D.T. (1963) Social attitudes and other acquired behavioural dispostitions, in S. Koch (ed.) *Psychology: A Study of a Science*, Vol. 6. New York: McGraw-Hill.

Campbell, M.C. (1999) Perceptions of price unfairness: antecedents and consequences, *Journal of Marketing Research*, 36: 187–99.

Campbell, M.C. and Kirmani, A. (2000) Consumers' use of persuasion knowledge: the effects of accessibility and cognitive capacity on perceptions of an influence agent, *Journal of Consumer Research*, 27: 69–83.

Cantor, J.R., Bryant, J. and Zillman, D. (1974) Enhancement of humor appreciation by transferred excitation, *Journal of Personality and Social Psychology*, 30: 812–21.

Capozza, D. and Bagozzi, R.P. (2001) Self-regulation in eating: the choice of traditional versus Mediterranean diets. Paper under review.

Carnegie-Mellon University Marketing Seminar (1978) Attitude change or attitude formation? An unanswered question, *Journal of Consumer Research*, 4: 271–6.

Carpenter, G.S., Glazer, R. and Nakamoto, K. (1994) Meaningful brands from meaningless differentiation: the dependence on irrelevant attributes, *Journal of Marketing Research*, 31: 339–50.

Carver, C.S. and Scheier, M.F. (1998) *On the Self-Regulation of Behavior*. Cambridge, UK: Cambridge University Press.

Chaiken, S. (1980) Heuristic versus systematic information processing and the use of source versus message cues in persuasion, *Journal of Personality and Social Psychology*, 39: 752–66.

Chaiken, S. and Trope, Y. (1999) *Dual Process Theories in Social Psychology*. New York: Guilford.

Childers, T.L. and Houston, M.J. (1984) Conditions for a picture-superiority effect on consumer memory, *Journal of Consumer Research*, 11: 643–54.

Chiu, L.H. (1972) A cross-cultural comparison of cognitive styles in Chinese and American children, *International Journal of Psychology*, 8: 235–42.

Clark, M.D. and Teasdale, J.D. (1982) Diurnal variation in clinical depression and accessibility of memories of positive and negative experiences, *Journal of Abnormal Psychology*, 91: 87–95.

Clore, G.L. and Byrne, D. (1974) A reinforcement affect model of attraction, in T.L. Huston (ed.) *Foundations of Interpersonal Attraction*. New York: Academic Press.

Clore, G.L., Schwarz, N. and Conway, M. (1994) Affective causes and consequences of social information processing, in R.S. Wyer and T.K. Srull (eds) *Handbook of Social Cognition*, 2nd edn, Vol. 1. Hillsdale, NJ: Erlbaum.

Cohen, J. (1978) Partialled products *are* interactions; partialled powers *are* curve components, *Psychological Bulletin*, 85: 858–66.

Cohen, J.B. and Areni, C.S. (1991) Affect and consumer behavior, in T.S. Robertson and H.H. Kassarjian (eds) *Handbook of Consumer Behavior*. Englewood Cliffs, NJ: Prentice-Hall.

Cohen, J.B. and Basu, K. (1987) Alternative models of categorization: toward a contingent processing framework, *Journal of Consumer Research*, 13: 455–72.

Cohen, J.B., Fishbein, M. and Ahtola, O.T. (1972) The nature and uses of expectancy-value models in consumer research, *Journal of Marketing Research*, 9: 456–60.

Cole, C.A. and Balasubramanian, S.K. (1993) Age differences in consumers' search for information: public policy implications, *Journal of Consumer Research*, 20: 157–69.

Collins, A.M. and Loftus, E.F. (1975) A spreading-activation theory of semantic processing, *Psychological Review*, 82: 407–28.

Conner, M. and Armitage, C.J. (1998) Extending the theory of planned behavior: a review and avenues for further research, *Journal of Applied Social Psychology*, 28: 1429–64.

Conner, M. and McMillan, B. (1999) Interaction effects in the theory of planned behaviour: studying cannabis use, *British Journal of Social Psychology*, 38: 195–222.

Conner, M. and Sparks, P. (1996) The theory of planned behaviour and health behaviours, in M. Conner and P. Norman (eds) *Predicting Health Behaviour: Research and Practive with Social Cognition Models*. Buckingham: Open University Press.

Cook, T.D. and Flay, B. (1978) The temporal persistence of experimentally induced attitude change: an evaluative review, in L. Berkowitz (ed.) *Advances in Experimental Social Psychology*, Vol. 11. New York: Academic Press.

Costley, C., Das, S. and Brucks, M. (1997) Presentation medium and spontaneous imaging effects on consumer memory, *Journal of Consumer Psychology*, 6: 211–32.

Crites, Jr, S.L., Fabrigar, L.R. and Retty, R.E. (1994) Measuring the affective and cognitive properties of attitudes: conceptual and methodological issues, *Personality and Social Psychology Bulletin*, 20: 619–34.

Dabholkar, P.A. (1999) Expectancy-value models, in P.E. Earl and S. Kemp (eds) *The Elgar Companion to Consumer Research and Economic Psychology*. Cheltenham: Edward Elgar.

Damasio, A.R. (1994) *Descartes' Error: Emotion, Reason, and the Human Brain*. New York: Avon.

Damasio, A.R. (1999) *The Feeling of What Happens: Body and Emotion in the Making of Consciousness*. New York: Harcourt Brace.

Davidson, A.R. and Morrison, D.M. (1983) Predicting contraceptive behavior from attitudes: a comparison of within- versus across-subjects procedures, *Journal of Personality and Social Psychology*, 45: 997–1009.

Davis, F.D., Bagozzi, R.P. and Warshaw, P.R. (1989) User acceptance of computer technology: a comparison of two theoretical models, *Management Science*, 35: 982–1003.

Davis, F.D., Bagozzi, R.P. and Warshaw, P.R. (1992) Extrinsic and intrinsic motivation to use computers in the workplace, *Journal of Applied Social Psychology*, 22: 1111–32.

Davis, W.A. (1984a) The two senses of desire, *Philosophical Studies*, 45: 181–95.

Davis, W.A. (1984b) A causal theory of intending, *American Philosophical Quarterly*, 21: 43–54.

Dawar, N. (1996) Extensions of broad brands: the role of retrieval in evaluations of fit, *Journal of Consumer Psychology*, 5: 189–207.

Dawar, N. and Pillutla, M.M. (2000) Impact of product-harm crises on brand equity: the moderating role of consumer expectations, *Journal of Marketing Research*, 37: 215–26.

DeFleur, M.L. and Westie, F.R. (1958) Verbal attitudes and overt acts: an experiment on the salience of attitudes, *American Sociological Review*, 23: 667–73.

Dholakia, U.M. and Bagozzi, R.P. (2001) Collaborative browsing and participation in virtual communities: a study of social interactions in digital environments. Unpublished working paper, Rice University.

Dholakia, U.M. and Bagozzi, R.P. (2002) As time goes by: how goal and implementation intentions influence enactment of short-fuse behaviors, *Journal of Applied Social Psychology*.

Dholakia, U.M., Bagozzi, R.P. and Nataraagan, R. (2001) The interplay of emotional and motivational influences on enactment of dissonant consumption impulses. Unpublished working paper, Rice University.

Diaz, R.M. and Berk, L.E. (1992) *Private Speech: From Social Interaction to Self-Regulation*. Hillsdale, NJ: Erlbaum.

Dick, A., Chakravarti, D. and Biehal, G. (1990) Memory-based inferences during consumer choice, *Journal of Consumer Research*, 17: 82–93.

Diener, E. and Emmons, R.A. (1985) The independence of positive and negative affect, *Journal of Personality and Social Psychology*, 47: 1105–17.

Diener, E. and Larsen, R.J. (1993) The experience of emotional well-being, in M. Lewis and J.M. Haviland (eds) *Handbook of Emotions*. New York: Guilford.

Dillon, W.R. and Kumar, A. (1985) Attitude organization and the attitude-behavior relation: a critique of Bagozzi and Burnkrant's reanalysis of Fishbein and Ajzen, *Journal of Personality and Social Psychology*, 49: 33–46.

Donovan, R.J. and Rossiter, J.R. (1982) Store atmospherics: an environmental psychology approach, *Journal of Retailing*, 58: 34–57.

Dubé, L., Bélanger, M-C. and Trudeau, E. (1996) The role of emotions in health care satisfaction, *Journal of Health Care Marketing*, 16: 45–51.

Dutton, D.G. and Aron, A.P. (1974) Some evidence for heightened sexual attraction under conditions of high anxiety, *Journal of Personality and Social Psychology*, 30: 510–17.

Dweck, C.S. (1991) Self-theories and goals: their role in motivation, personality, and development, in R. Dienstbier (ed.) *Nebraska Symposium on Motivation*, Vol. 38. Lincoln, NE: University of Nebraska Press.

Eagly, A.H. and Chaiken, S. (1993) *The Psychology of Attitudes*. Fort Worth, TX: Harcourt Brace Jovanovich.

Eagly, A.H., Mladinic, C. and Otto, S. (1994) Cognitive and affective bases of attitudes toward social groups and social policies, *Journal of Experimental Social Psychology*, 30: 113–37.

East, R. (1997) *Consumer Behavior: Advances and Applications in Marketing*. London: Prentice-Hall.

Edell, J.A. and Burke, M.C. (1987) The power of feelings in understanding advertising effects, *Journal of Consumer Research*, 14: 421–33.

Edell, J.A. and Staelin, R. (1983) The information processing of pictures in print advertisements, *Journal of Consumer Research*, 10: 45–61.

Edwards, W. (1954) The theory of decision making, *Psychological Bulletin*, 51: 380–417.

Eich, E.J. and Birnbaum, I.M. (1982) Repetition, cueing and state-dependent memory, *Memory and Cognition*, 10: 103–14.

Ekman, P. (1993) Facial expression and emotion, *American Psychologist*, 48: 384–92.

Ellemers, N., Kortekaas, P. and Ouwekerk, J. (1999) Self-categorisation, commitment to the group and group self-esteem as related but distinct aspects of social identity, *European Journal of Social Psychology*, 29: 371–89.

Elms, A.C. (1966) Influence of fantasy ability on attitude change through role-playing, *Journal of Personality and Social Psychology*, 4: 36–43.

Engel, J.F., Blackwell, R.D. and Miniard, P.W. (1995) *Consumer Behavior*, 8th edn. New York: Dryden.

Erber, R. and Fiske, S.T. (1984) Outcome dependency and attention to inconsistent information, *Journal of Personality and Social Psychology*, 47: 709–26.

Evans, M.G. (1991) The problem of analyzing multivariate composites: interactions revisited, *American Psychologist*, 46: 6–15.

Fazio, R.H. (1986) How do attitudes guide behavior?, in R.M. Sorrentino and E.T. Higgins (eds) *Handbook of Social Behavior*. New York: Guilford.

Fazio, R.H. (1989) On the power and functionality of attitudes: the role of attitude accessibility, in A.R. Pratkanis, S.J. Breckler and A.G. Greenwald (eds) *Attitude Structure and Function*. Hillsdale, NJ: Erlbaum.

Fazio, R.H. (1990) Multiple processes by which attitudes guide behavior: the MODE model as an integrative framework, in M.P. Zanna (ed.) *Advances in Experimental Social Psychology*, Vol. 23. San Diego, CA: Academic Press.

Fazio, R.H. (1995) Attitudes as object-evaluation associations: determinants, consequences, and correlates of attitude accessibility, in R.E. Petty and J.A. Krosnik (eds) *Attitude Strength: Antecedents and Consequences*. Mahway, NJ: Erlbaum.

Fazio, R.H. and Powell, M.C. (1997) On the value of knowing one's likes and dislikes: attitude accessibility, stress, and health in college, *Psychological Science*, 8: 430–6.

Fazio, R.H. and Williams, C.J. (1986) Attitude accessibility as a moderator of the attitude–perception and attitude–behavior relations: an investigation of the 1984 presidential election, *Journal of Personality and Social Psychology*, 51: 505–14.

Fazio, R.H., Zanna, M.P. and Cooper, J. (1977) Dissonance and self-perception: An integrative view of each theory's proper domain of application, *Journal of Experimental Social Psychology*, 13: 464–79.

Fazio, R.H., Powell, M.C. and Herr, P.M. (1983) Toward a process model of the attitude–behavior relation: accessing one's attitude upon mere observation of the attitude object, *Journal of Personality and Social Psychology*, 44: 723–35.

Fazio, R.H., Powell, M. and Williams, C.J. (1989) The role of attitude accessibility in the attitude-to-behavior process, *Journal of Consumer Research*, 16: 280–8.

Fazio, R.H., Blascovich, J. and Driscoll, D.M. (1992a) On the functional value of attitudes: the influence of accessible attitudes upon the ease and quality of decision making, *Personality and Social Psychology Bulletin*, 18: 339–57.

Fazio, R.H., Herr, P.M. and Powell, M.C. (1992b) On the development and strength of category-brand associations in memory: the case of mystery ads, *Journal of Consumer Psychology*, 1: 1–13.

Fazio, R., Ledbetter, J. and Towles-Schwen, T. (2000) On the costs of accessible attitudes: detecting that the attitude object has changed, *Journal of Personality and Social Psychology*, 78: 197–210.

Feather, N.T. (1982) Expectancy value approaches: present status and future directions, in N.T. Feather (ed.) *Expectations and Actions: Expectancy Value Models in Psychology*. Hillsdale, NJ: Erlbaum.

Feldman, J.M. and Lynch, J.G. (1988) Self-generated validity and other effects of measurement of belief, attitude, intention, and behavior, *Journal of Applied Psychology*, 73: 421–35.

Festinger, L. (1957) *A Theory of Cognitive Dissonance*. Evanston, IL: Row, Peterson.

Festinger, L. (1964) *Conflict, Decision and Dissonance*. Stanford, CA: Stanford University Press.

Festinger, L. and Carlsmith, J.M. (1959) Cognitive consequences of forced compliance, *Journal of Abnormal and Social Psychology*, 58: 203–10.

Fiedler, K. (1990) Mood-dependent selectivity in social cognition, in W. Stroebe and M. Hewstone (eds) *European Review of Social Psychology*, Vol. 1. New York: Wiley.

Fishbein, M. (1967a) A consideration of beliefs, and their role in attitude measurement, in M. Fishbein (ed.) *Readings in Attitude Theory and Measurement*. New York: Wiley.

Fishbein, M. (1967b) A behavior theory approach to the relations between beliefs about an object and the attitude toward the object, in M. Fishbein (ed.) *Readings in Attitude Theory and Measurement*. New York: Wiley.

Fishbein, M. (1980) A theory of reasoned action: some applications and implications, in H.E. Howe Jr and M.M. Page (eds) *Nebraska Symposium on Motivation 1979: Beliefs, Attitudes and Values*. Lincoln, NE: University of Nebraska Press.

Fishbein, M. (1993) Introduction by Martin Fishbein, in D.J. Terry, C. Gallois and M. McCamish (eds) *The Theory of Reasoned Action: Its Application to AIDS-Preventive Behaviour*. Oxford: Pergamon.

Fishbein, M. and Ajzen, I. (1975) *Belief, Attitude, Intention, and Behavior: An Introduction to Theory and Research*. Reading, MA: Addison-Wesley.

Fishbein, M. and Ajzen, I. (1981) Acceptance, yielding, and impact: cognitive processes in persuasion, in R. Petty, T. Ostrom and T. Brock (eds) *Cognitive Responses in Persuasion*. Hillsdale, NJ: Erlbaum.

Fishbein, M. and Stasson, M. (1990) The role of desires, self-predictions, and perceived control in the prediction of training session attendance, *Journal of Applied Social Psychology*, 20: 173–98.

Fiske, S.T. and Neuberg, S.L. (1990) A continuum of impression formation, from category-based to individuating processes: influences of information and motivation on attention and interpretation, in M.P. Zanna (ed.) *Advances in Experimental Social Psychology*, Vol. 23. New York: Academic Press.

Fiske, S.T. and Pavelchak, M.A. (1986) Category-based versus piecemeal-based affective responses: developments in schema-triggered affect, in R.M. Sorrentino and E.T. Higgings (eds) *Handbook of Motivation and Cognition: Foundations of Social Behaviour*. New York: Guilford.

Fiske, S.T. and Taylor, S.E. (1991) *Social Cognition*, 2nd edn. New York: McGraw-Hill.

Fleming, D. (1967) Attitude: the history of a concept, *Perspectives in American History*, 1: 285–365.

Fleming, M.A. and Petty, R.E. (1999) Identity and persuasion: an elaboration likelihood approach, in M.A. Hogg and D.J. Terry (eds) *Attitudes, Behavior, and Social Context: The Role of Norms and Group Membership*. Mahwah, NJ: Erlbaum.

Folkes, V.S. (1984) Consumer reactions to product failure: an attributional approach, *Journal of Consumer Research*, 10: 398–409.

Folkes, V.S. (1988) Recent attribution research in consumer behavior: a review and new directions, *Journal of Consumer Research*, 14: 548–65.

Folkes, V.S. and Kamins, M.A. (1999) Effects of information about firms' ethical and unethical actions on consumers' attitudes, *Journal of Consumer Psychology*, 8: 243–60.

Folkes, V.S. and Kiesler, T. (1991) Social cognition: consumers' inferences about the self and others, in T.S. Robertson and H.H. Kassarjian (eds) *Handbook of Consumer Behavior*. Englewood Cliffs, NJ: Prentice-Hall.

Folkes, V., Koletsky, S. and Graham, J.L. (1987) A field study of causal inferences and consumer reaction: the view from the airport, *Journal of Consumer Research*, 13: 534–9.

Folkes, V.S., Martin, I.M. and Gupta, K. (1993) When to say when: effects of supply on usage, *Journal of Consumer Research*, 20: 467–77.

Forgas, J.P. (1994) The role of emotion in social judgments: an introductory review and an affect infusion model (AIM), *European Journal of Social Psychology*, 24: 1–24.

Forgas, J.P. (1995) Mood and judgment: the affect infusion model (AIM), *Psychological Bulletin*, 117(1): 39–66.

Forgas, J.P. and Bower, G.H. (1987) Mood effects on person-perception judgments, *Journal of Personality and Social Psychology*, 53(1): 53–60.

Fournier, S. (1998) Consumers and their brands: developing relationship theory in consumer research, *Journal of Consumer Research*, 24: 343–73.

Foxall, G.R. (1996) *Consumers in Context: The BPM Research Program*. London: ITP.

Foxall, G.R. (1997) *Marketing Psychology: The Paradigm in the Wings*. London: Macmillan.

Frankfurt, H. (1988) *The Importance of What We Care about*. Cambridge, UK: Cambridge University Press.

Fredericks, A.J. and Dossett, D.L. (1983) Attitude–behavior relations: a comparison of the Fishbein-Ajzen and the Bentler-Speckart models, *Journal of Personality and Social Psychology*, 45: 501–12.

Friedman, A. and Polson, M.C. (1981) Hemispheres as independent resource system: limited-capacity processing and cerebral specialization, *Journal of Experimental Psychology*, 7: 1031–58.

Friestad, M. and Thorson, E. (1986) Emotion-eliciting advertising: effect on long-term memory and judgment, *Advances in Consumer Research*, 13: 111–15.

Frijda, N.H. (1986) *The Emotions*. Cambridge: Cambridge University Press.

Frijda, N.H. (1987) Emotion, cognitive structure, and action tendency, *Cognition and Emotion*, 1: 115–43.

Frijda, N.H. (1993) Moods, emotion episodes, and emotions, in M.L. Haviland and J.M. Haviland (eds) *Handbook of Emotions*. New York: Guilford.

Frijda, N.H. (1994) Emotions are functional, most of the time, in P. Ekman and R.J. Davidson (eds) *The Nature of Emotion*. New York: Oxford University Press.

Frijda, N.H., Kuipers, P. and ter Shure, E. (1989) Relations among emotion, appraisal, and emotional action readiness, *Journal of Personality and Social Psychology*, 57: 212–28.

Gaither, C.A., Bagozzi, R.P., Ascione, F.J. and Kirking, D.M. (1996) A reasoned action approach to physician's utilization of drug information sources, *Pharmaceutical Research*, 13: 1291–8.

Gaither, C.A., Bagozzi, R.P., Ascione, F.J. and Kirking, D.M. (1997) The determinants of physician attitudes and subjective norms toward drug information sources: modification and test of the theory of reasoned action, *Pharmaceutical Research*, 14: 1298–308.

Garbarino, E. and Johnson, M. (1999) The different roles of satisfaction, trust, and commitment in customer relationships, *Journal of Marketing*, 63: 70–87.

Gardner, M.P. (1985) Mood states and consumer behavior: a critical review, *Journal of Consumer Research*, 12: 281–300.

Gardner, M.P. and Simokos, G.J. (1986) Toward a methodology for assessing effects of instore atmospherics, *Advances in Consumer Research*, 13: 27–31.

Gelman, S.A. and Markman, E.M. (1986) Categories and induction in young children, *Cognition*, 23: 183–209.

Gensch, D.H. and Svestka, J.A. (1984) A maximum likelihood hierarchical disaggregate model for predicting choices of individuals, *Journal of Mathematical Psychology*, 28: 160–78.

Gleicher, F., Boninger, D.S., Neter, E. et al. (1994) The use of counterfactual simulation to change attitudes about safe sex. Unpublished raw data, reported in Gleicher et al. (1995).

Gleicher, F., Boninger, D.S., Strathman, A. et al. (1995) With an eye toward the future: the impact of counterfactual thinking on affect, attitudes, and behavior, in N.J. Roese and J.M. Olson (eds) *What Might Have Been: The Social Psychology of Counterfactual Thinking*. Mahwah, NJ: Erlbaum.

Gold, M. with Douvan, E. (1997) *A New Outline of Social Psychology*. Washington, DC: American Psychological Association.

Goldberg, M.E. and Gorn, G.J. (1987) Happy and sad TV programs: how they affect reactions to commercials, *Journal of Consumer Research*, 14: 387–403.

Gollwitzer, P.M. (1996) The volitional benefits of planning, in P.M. Gollwitzer and J.A. Bargh (eds) *The Psychology of Action: Linking Cognition and Motivation to Behavior*. New York: Guilford.

Gollwitzer, P.M. and Brandstätter, V. (1997) Implementation intentions and effective goal pursuit, *Journal of Personality and Social Psychology*, 73: 186–99.

Gollwitzer, P.M., Heckhausen, H. and Stellar, B. (1990) Deliberative and implemental mind-sets: cognitive tuning toward congrous thoughts and information, *Journal of Personality and Social Psychology*, 59: 1119–27.

Goodstein, R.C. (1993) Category-based applications and extensions in advertising: motivating more extensive ad processing, *Journal of Consumer Research*, 20: 87–99.

Gopinath, M. and Bagozzi, R.P. (2001) Cognitive appraisals leading to consumer emotions and action tendencies. Unpublished working paper, University of Michigan.

Gorn, G.J., Chattopadhyay, A., Yi, T. and Dahl, D.W. (1997) Effects of color as an executional cue in advertising: they're in the shade, *Management Science*, 43(10): 1387–400.

Goschke, T. and Kuhl, J. (1996) Remembering what to do: explicit and implicit memory for intentions, in M. Brandimonte, G.O. Einstein and M.A. McDaniel (eds) *Prospective Memory: Theory and Applications*. Mahwah, NJ: Erlbaum.

Green, D.P., Goldman, S.L. and Salovey, P. (1993) Measurement error masks bipolarity in affect ratings, *Journal of Personality and Social Psychology*, 64: 1029–41.

Green, P.E. and Krieger, A.M. (1992) An application of a product positioning model to pharmaceutical products, *Marketing Science*, 11: 117–32.

Green, P.E. and Srinivasan, V. (1990) Conjoint analysis in marketing research: new developments and directions, *Journal of Marketing*, 54: 3–19.

Green, P.E., Krieger, A.M. and Agarwal, M.K. (1993) A cross validation test of four models for quantifying multiattribute preferences, *Marketing Letters*, 4: 369–80.

Greenleaf, E.A. (1995) The impact of reference price effects on the profitability of price promotions, *Marketing Science*, 14: 82–104.

Greenwald, A.G. (1968) Cognitive learning, cognitive response to persuasion, and attitude change, in A. Greenwald, T. Brock and T. Ostrom (eds) *Psychological Foundations of Attitudes*. New York: Academic Press.

Greenwald, A.G. (1975) On the inconclusiveness of 'crucial' cognitive tests of dissonance versus self-perception theories, *Journal of Experimental Social Psychology*, 11: 490–9.

Greenwald, A.G. and Banaji, M.R. (1995) Implicit social cognition: attitudes, self-esteem, and stereotypes, *Psychological Review*, 102: 4–27.

Greenwald, A.G., Brock, T.C. and Ostrom, T. (1968) *Psychological Foundations of Attitudes*. New York: Academic Press.

Gregan-Paxton, J. and John, D.R. (1997) The emergence of adaptive decision making in children, *Journal of Consumer Research*, 24: 43–56.

Griffin, A. and Hauser, J.R. (1993) The voice of the customer, *Marketing Science*, 12: 1–27.

Gürhan-Canli, Z. and Maheswaran, D. (1998) The effects of extensions on brand name dilution and enhancement, *Journal of Marketing Research*, 35: 464–73.

Gürhan-Canli, Z. and Maheswaran, D. (2000) Determinants of country-of-origin evaluations, *Journal of Consumer Research*, 27: 96–108.

Gutman, J. (1982) A means-end chain model based on consumer categorization processes, *Journal of Marketing*, 46: 60–72.

Haddock, G. and Zanna, M.P. (1998) On the use of open-ended measures to assess attitudinal components, *British Journal of Social Psychology*, 37: 129–49.

Hamilton, D.L., Driscoll, D.M. and Worth, L.T. (1989) Cognitive organization of impressions: effects of incongruency in complex representations, *Journal of Personality and Social Psychology*, 57: 925–39.

Hansen, F. (1981) Hemispheral lateralization: implications for understanding consumer behavior, *Journal of Consumer Research*, 8: 23–36.

Harkins, S.G. and Petty, R.E. (1981) The effects of source magnification of cognitive effort on attitudes: an information processing view, *Journal of Personality and Social Psychology*, 40: 401–13.

Harkins, S.G. and Petty, R.E. (1987) Information utility and the multiple source effect, *Journal of Personality and Social Psychology*, 52: 260–8.

Harré, R. and Stearns, P. (1995) *Discursive Psychology in Practice*. London: Sage.

Hastie, R. and Park, B. (1986) The relationship between memory and judgment depends on whether the judgment task is memory-based or on-line, *Psychological Review*, 93: 258–68.

Haugtvedt, C.P. and Petty, R.E. (1992) Personality and persuasion: need for cognition moderates the persistence and resistance of attitude changes, *Journal of Personality and Social Psychology*, 63: 308–19.

Haugtvedt, C.P. and Wegener, D.T. (1994) Message order effects in persuasion: an attitude strength perspective, *Journal of Consumer Research*, 21: 205–18.

Hawkins, S.A. and Hoch, S.J. (1992) Low-involvement learning: memory without evaluation, *Journal of Consumer Research*, 19: 212–25.

Hayes-Roth, B. (1977) Evolution of cognitive structures and processes, *Psychological Review*, 84: 260–78.

Heckler, S.E. and Childers, T.L. (1992) The role of expectancy and relevancy in memory for verbal and visual information: what is incongruency?, *Journal of Consumer Research*, 18: 475–92.

Heider, F. (1958) *The Psychology of Interpersonal Relations*. New York: Wiley.

Helson, H. (1964) *Adaptation-Level Theory*. New York: Harper and Row.

Herr, P.M. (1986) Consequences of priming: judgment and behavior, *Journal of Personality and Social Psychology*, 51: 1106–15.

Herr, P.M. (1989) Priming price: prior knowledge and context effects, *Journal of Consumer Research*, 16: 67–75.

Herr, P.B., Sherman, S.J. and Fazio, R.H. (1983) On the consequences of priming: assimilation and contrast effects, *Journal of Experimental Social Psychology*, 19: 323–40.

Herr, P.M., Kardes, F.R. and Kim, J. (1991) Effects of word-of-mouth and product-attribute information on persuasion: an accessibility-diagnosticity perspective, *Journal of Consumer Research*, 17: 454–62.

Herr, P.M., Farquhar, P.H. and Fazio, R.H. (1996) Impact of dominance and relatedness on brand extensions, *Journal of Consumer Psychology*, 5: 135–59.

Hewstone, M., Johnston, L. and Aird, P. (1992) Cognitive models of stereotype change: (2) Perceptions of homogeneous and heterogeneous groups, *European Journal of Social Psychology*, 22: 235–49.

Hewstone, M., Macrae, C.N., Griffiths, R. and Milne, A.B. (1994) Cognitive models of stereotype change: (5) Measurement, development, and consequences of subtyping, *Journal of Experimental Social Psychology*, 30: 505–26.

Higgins, E.T. (1996) Knowledge activation: accessibility, applicability, and salience, in E.T. Higgins and A.W. Kruglanski (eds) *Social Psychology: Handbook of Basic Principles*. New York: Guilford.

Higgins, E.T., King, G.A. and Mavin, G.H. (1982) Individual construct accessibility and subjective impressions and recall, *Journal of Personality and Social Psychology*, 43: 35–47.

Hill, R.P. and Gardner, M.P. (1987) The buying process: effects of and on consumer mood states, *Advances in Consumer Research*, 14: 408–10.

Hinsz, V.B. and Ployhart, R.E. (1998) Trying, intentions, and the processes by which goals influence performance: an empirical test of the theory of goal pursuit, *Journal of Applied Social Psychology*, 28: 1051–66.

Hochschild, A.R. (1983) *The Managed Heart*. Berkeley, CA: University of California Press.

Hoffman, M.L. (2000) *Empathy and Moral Development: Implications for Caring and Justice*. Cambridge: Cambridge University Press.

Hogg, M.A. and Abrams, D. (1988) *Social Identification: A Social Psychology of Intergroup Relations and Group Processes*. London: Routledge.

Holbrook, M.B. and Batra, R. (1987) Assessing the role of emotions as mediators of consumer responses to advertising, *Journal of Consumer Research*, 14: 404–20.

Honderich, T. (ed.) (1995) *The Oxford Companion to Philosophy*. Oxford: Oxford University Press.

Hong, S-T. and Wyer, R.S. (1989) Effects of country-of-origin and product-attribute information on product evaluation: an information processing perspective, *Journal of Consumer Research*, 16: 175–87.

Hong, S-T. and Wyer, R.S. (1990) Determinants of product evaluation: effects of the time interval between knowledge of a product's country of origin and information about its specific attributes, *Journal of Consumer Research*, 17: 277–88.

Hornik, J. (1992) Tactile stimulation and consumer response, *Journal of Consumer Research*, 19: 449–58.

Hornsby, J. (1980) *Actions*. London: Routledge and Kegan Paul.

Houston, D.A. and Fazio, R.H. (1989) Biased processing as a function of attitude accessibility: making objective judgments subjectively, *Social Cognition*, 7: 51–66.

Houston, M.J., Childers, T.L. and Heckler, S.E. (1987) Picture-word consistency and the elaborative processing of advertisements, *Journal of Marketing Research*, 24: 359–69.

Hovland, C.I. (1951) Human learning and retention, in S.S. Stevens (ed.) *Handbook of Experimental Psychology*. New York: Wiley.

Hovland, C.I. (1957) *The Order of Presentation in Persuasion*. New Haven, CT: Yale University Press.

Hovland, C.I. and Janis, I.L. (1959) *Personality and Persuasability*. New Haven, CT: Yale University Press.

Hovland, C.I. and Rosenberg, M.J. (1960) *Attitude Organization and Change: An Analysis of Consistency among Attitude Components*. New Haven, CT: Yale University Press.

Hovland, C.I. and Weiss, W. (1951) The influence of source credibility on communication effectiveness, *Public Opinion Quarterly*, 15: 635–50.

Hovland, C.I., Lumsdaine, A.A. and Sheffield, A.A. (1949) *Experiments on Mass Communication*. Princeton, NJ: Princeton University Press.

Hovland, C.I., Janis, I.L. and Kelley, H.H. (1953) *Communication and Persuasion: Psychological Studies of Opinion Change*. New Haven, CT: Yale University Press.

Hoyer, W.D. and MacInnis, D.J. (2001) *Consumer Behavior*, 2nd edn. Boston, MA: Houghton Mifflin.

Hoyer, W.D., Srivastava, R.K. and Jacoby, J. (1984) Sources of miscomprehension in television advertising, *Journal of Advertising*, 13: 17–27.

Huber, J. and McCann, J. (1982) The impact of inferential beliefs on product evaluations, *Journal of Marketing Research*, 19: 324–33.

Hutchinson, J.W. and Moore, D.L. (1984) Issues surrounding the examination of delay effects of advertising, in T.C. Kinnear (ed.) *Advances in Consumer Research*, Vol. 2. Provo, UT: Association for Consumer Research.

Insko, C.A. (1984) Balance theory, the Jordan paradigm, and the Wiest tetrahedron, in L. Berkowitz (ed.) *Advances in Experimental Social Psychology*, Vol. 18. San Diego, CA: Academic Press.

Isen, A.M. (1984) Toward understanding the role of affect in cognition, in R.S. Wyer and T.K. Srull (eds) *Handbook of Social Cognition*, Vol. 3. Hillsdale, NJ: Erlbaum.

Isen, A.M. (1987) Positive affect, cognitive processes, and social behavior, in L. Berkowitz (ed.) *Advances in Experimental Social Psychology*, Vol. 20. New York: Academic Press.

Isen, A.M. (1989) Some ways in which affect influences cognitive processes: implications for advertising and consumer behavior, in P. Cafferata and A.M. Tybout (eds) *Cognitive and Affective Responses to Advertising*. Lexington, MA: Lexington Books.

Isen, A.M. and Daubman, K.A. (1984) The influence of affect on categorization, *Journal of Personality and Social Psychology*, 47: 1206–17.

Isen, A.M., Shalker, T.E., Clark, M. and Karp, L. (1978) Affect, accessibility of material in memory, and behavior: a cognitive loop? *Journal of Personality and Social Psychology*, 36: 1–12.

Isen, A.M., Johnson, M.M., Mertz, E. and Robinson, G.F. (1985) The influence of positive affect on the unusualness of word associations, *Journal of Personality and Social Psychology*, 48: 1–14.

Isen, A.M., Daubman, K.A. and Nowicki, G.P. (1987) Positive affect facilitates creative problem solving, *Journal of Personality and Social Psychology*, 52: 1122–31.

Isen, A.M., Niedenthal, P.M. and Cantor, N. (1992) An influence of positive affect on social categorization, *Motivation and Emotion*, 16: 65–78.

Izard, C.E. (1972) *Patterns of Emotions: A New Analysis of Anxiety and Depression*. New York: Academic Press.

Izard, C.E. (1991) *The Psychology of Emotions*. New York: Plenum.

Izard, C.E. (1992) Basic emotions, relations among emotions, and emotion–cognition relations, *Psychological Review*, 99: 561–5.

Jacoby, J. and Hoyer, W.D. (1987) *The Comprehension and Miscomprehension of Print Communications: An Investigation of Mass Media Magazines*. New York: Erlbaum.

Jacoby, J., Jaccard, J.J., Currim, I., Kuss, A., Ansari, A. and Troutman, T. (1994) Tracing the impact of item-by-item information accessing on uncertainty reduction, *Journal of Consumer Research*, 21: 291–303.

James, W. (1890) *The Principles of Psychology*, Vol. 2. New York: Holt (reprinted by Dover Publications, New York, 1950).

Janiszewski, C. (1988) Preconscious processing effect: the independence of attitude formation and conscious thought, *Journal of Consumer Research*, 15: 199–209.

Janiszewski, C. (1990) The influence of print advertisement organization on affect toward a brand name, *Journal of Consumer Research*, 17: 53–65.

Janiszewski, C. (1993) Preattentive mere exposure effects, *Journal of Consumer Research*, 20: 376–92.

Janiszewski, C. (1998) The influence of display characteristics on visual exploratory search behavior, *Journal of Consumer Research*, 25: 290–301.

Janiszewski, C. and Lichtenstein, D.R. (1999) A range theory account of price perception, *Journal of Consumer Research*, 25: 353–68.

Jaspers, J.M.G. (1978) Determinants of attitude and attitude change, in H. Taijfel and C. Fraser (eds) *Introducing Social Psychology*. Harmondsworth: Penguin.

Johar, G.V. (1995) Involvement and deception from implied advertising claims, *Journal of Marketing Research*, 32: 267–79.

Johar, G.V. and Pham, M.T. (1999) Relatedness, prominence, and constructive sponsor identification, *Journal of Marketing Research*, 36: 299–312.

Johar, G.V. and Simmons, C.J. (2000) The use of concurrent disclosures to correct invalid inferences, *Journal of Consumer Research*, 26: 307–22.

John, D.R. and Sujan, M. (1990) Age differences in product categorization, *Journal of Consumer Research*, 16: 452–60.

John, D.R., Scott, C.A. and Bettman, J.R. (1986) Sampling data for covariation assessment: the effect of prior beliefs on search patterns, *Journal of Consumer Research*, 13: 38–47.

Johnson, B.T. and Eagly, A.H. (1989) Effects on involvement on persuasion: a meta-analysis, *Psychological Bulletin*, 106: 290–314.

Johnson, H.H. and Watkins, T.A. (1971) The effects of message repetition on immediate and delayed attitude change, *Psychonomic Science*, 22: 101–3.

Johnson, M.D. (1998) *Customer Orientation and Market Action*. Upper Saddle River, NJ: Prentice-Hall.

Johnson, M.D. and Gustafsson, A. (2000) *Improving Customer Satisfaction, Loyalty and Profit: An Integrated Measurement and Management System*. San Francisco, CA: Jossey-Bass.

Johnson, M.K., Hashtroudi, S. and Lindsay, D.S. (1993) Source monitoring, *Psychological Bulletin*, 114: 3–28.

Johnson, R.D. and Levin, I.P. (1985) More than meets the eye: the effect of missing information on purchase evaluations, *Journal of Consumer Research*, 12: 169–77.

Johnston, L. and Hewstone, M. (1992) Cognitive models of stereotype change: (3) Subtyping and the perceived typicality of disconfirming group members, *Journal of Experimental Social Psychology*, 28: 360–86.

Joiner, C. and Loken, B. (1998) The inclusion effect and category-based induction: theory and application to brand categories, *Journal of Consumer Psychology*, 7: 101–30.

Kahn, B.E. and Isen, A.M. (1993) The influence of positive affect on variety seeking among safe, enjoyable products, *Journal of Consumer Research*, 20: 257–71.

Kahneman, D. (1973) *Attention and Effort*. Englewood Cliffs, NJ: Prentice-Hall.

Kahneman, D. and Tversky, A. (1982) The simulation heuristic, in D. Kahneman, P. Slovic and A. Tversky (eds) *Judgment under Uncertainty: Heuristics and Biases*. New York: Cambridge University Press.

Kallgren, C.A. and Wood, W. (1986) Access to attitude-relevant information in memory as a determinant of attitude-behavior consistency, *Journal of Experimental Social Psychology*, 22: 328–38.

Kalyanaram, G. and Winer, R.S. (1995) Empirical generalizations from reference price research, *Marketing Science*, 14: 151–69.

Kardes, F.R. (1988) Spontaneous inference processes in advertising: the effects of conclusion omission and involvement on persuasion, *Journal of Consumer Research*, 15: 225–33.

Kardes, F.R. (1993) Consumer inference: determinants, consequences, and implications for advertising, in A.A. Mitchell (ed.) *Advertising Exposure, Memory and Choice*. Hillsdale, NJ: Erlbaum.

Kardes, F.R. (1999) *Consumer Behavior and Managerial Decision Making*. Reading, MA: Addison-Wesley.

Kardes, F.R. and Kalyanaram, G. (1992) Order-of-entry effects on consumer memory and judgement: an information integration perspective, *Journal of Marketing Research*, 29: 343–57.

Kardes, F.R., Kalyanaram, G., Chandrashekaran, M. and Dornoff, R.J. (1993) Brand retrieval, consideration set composition, consumer choice, and the pioneer advantage, *Journal of Consumer Research*, 20 (June): 62–75.

Katz, D. and Stotland, E. (1959) A preliminary statement to a theory of attitude structure and change, in S. Koch (ed.) *Psychology: A Study of a Science*, Vol. 3. New York: McGraw-Hill.

Keller, K.L. (1987) Memory factors in advertising: the effect of advertising retrieval cues on brand evaluations, *Journal of Consumer Research*, 14: 316–33.

Keller, K.L. (1991a) Cue compatibility and framing in advertising, *Journal of Marketing Research*, 28: 42–57.

Keller, K.L. (1991b) Memory and evaluation effects in competitive advertising environments, *Journal of Consumer Research*, 17: 463–76.

Keller, K.L. and Aaker, D.A. (1992) The effects of sequential introduction of brand extensions, *Journal of Marketing Research*, 29: 35–50.

Kelman, H.C. and Hovland, C.I. (1953) 'Reinstatement' of the communicator in delayed measurement of opinion change, *Journal of Abnormal and Social Psychology*, 48: 327–35.

Kent, R.J. and Allen, C.T. (1994) Competitive interference effects in consumer memory for advertising: the role of brand familiarity, *Journal of Marketing*, 58: 97–105.

Kiesler, C.A. and Munson, P.A. (1975) Attitudes and opinions, *Annual Review of Psychology*, 26: 415–56.

Kirmani, A. (1990) The effect of perceived advertising costs on brand perceptions, *Journal of Consumer Research*, 17: 160–71.

Klein, J.G., Ettenson, R. and Morris, M.D. (1998) The animosity model of foreign product purchase: an empirical test in the People's Republic of China, *Journal of Marketing*, 62: 89–100.

Klenosky, D.B., Gengler, C.E. and Mulvey, M.S. (1993) Understanding factors influencing ski destination choices: a means-end analytic approach, *Journal of Leisure Research*, 25: 362–79.

Kothandapani, V. (1971) Validation of feeling, belief, and intention to act as three components of attitude and their contribution to prediction of contraceptive behavior, *Journal of Personality and Social Psychology*, 19: 321–33.

Krech, D. and Crutchfield, R.S. (1948) *Theory and Problems of Social Psychology.* New York: McGraw-Hill.

Kruglanski, A.W. and Thompson, E.P. (1999) Persuasion by a single route: a view from the unimodel, *Psychological Inquiry*, 10: 83–109.

Kruglanski, A.W., Thompson, E.P. and Spiegel, S. (1999) Separate or equal? Bimodal notions of persuasion and a single-process 'Unimodel', in S. Chaiken and Y. Trope (eds) *Dual-Process Theories in Social Psychology.* New York: Guilford.

Kuhl, J. (1984) Motivational aspects of achievement motivation and learned helplessness: toward a comprehensive theory of action control, in B.A. Maher and W.B. Maher (eds) *Progress in Experimental Personality Research*, Vol. 13. New York: Academic Press.

Kuhl, J. and Beckmann, J. (1994) *Volition and Personality.* Toronto: Hogrefe.

Kumar, A. (2000) Interference effects of contextual cues in advertisements on memory for ad content, *Journal of Consumer Psychology*, 9: 155–66.

Kunda, Z. (1999) Parallel processing of stereotypes and behaviors, in S. Chaiken and Y. Trope (eds) *Dual-Process Theories in Social Psychology.* New York: Guilford.

Kutner, B., Wilkins, C. and Yarrow, P.R. (1952) Verbal attitudes and overt behavior involving racial prejudice, *Journal of Abnormal and Social Psychology*, 47: 649–52.

Kvavilashvili, L. and Ellis, J. (1996) Varieties of intention: some distinctions and classifications, in M. Brandimonte, G.O. Einstein and M.A. McDaniel (eds) *Prospective Memory: Theory and Applications.* Mahwah, NJ: Erlbaum.

Laird, J.D., Wagener, J.J., Halal, M. and Szegda, M. (1982) Remembering what you feel: the effects of emotion on memory, *Journal of Personality and Social Psychology*, 42(4): 646–57.

LaPierre, R.T. (1934) Attitudes versus actions, *Social Forces*, 13: 230–7.

Larsen, R.J. and Diener, E. (1992) Promises and problems with the circumplex model of emotion, in M.S. Clark (ed.) *Review of Personality and Social Psychology: Emotional and Social Behavior*, Vol. 14. Newbury Park, CA: Sage.

Law, S., Hawkins, S.A. and Craik, F.I.M. (1998) Repetition-induced belief in the elderly: rehabilitating age-related memory deficits, *Journal of Consumer Research*, 25: 91–107.

Lawson, R. (1997) Consumer decision making within a goal-driven framework, *Psychology & Marketing*, 14: 427–49.

Lazarus, R.S. (1982) Thoughts on the relations between emotion and cognition, *American Psychologist*, 35: 1019–24.

Lazarus, R.S. (1991) *Emotion and Adaptation*. New York: Oxford University Press.

LeDoux, J. (1996) *The Emotional Brain: The Mysterious Underpinnings of Emotional Life*. New York: Simon & Schuster.

Lee, A.Y. and Sternthal, B. (1999) The effects of positive mood on memory, *Journal of Consumer Research*, 26: 115–27.

Lee, H., Herr, P.M., Kim, C. and Kardes, F.R. (1999) Motivated search: effects of choice accountability, issue involvement, and prior knowledge on information acquisition and use, *Journal of Business Research*, 45: 75–88.

Leone, L. and Perugini, M. (2000) Tentare di studiare (Trying to study), *Giornale Italiano di Psicologia*, 4: 757–88.

Leone, L., Perugini, M. and Ercolani, A.P. (1999) A comparison of three models of attitude-behaviour relationships in studying behaviour domain, *European Journal of Social Psychology*, 29: 161–89.

Lewan, P.C. and Stotland, E. (1961) The effects of prior information on susceptibility to an emotional appeal, *Journal of Abnormal and Social Psychology*, 62: 450–3.

Lewis, M. (1993) Self-conscious emotions: embarrassment, pride, shame, and guilt, in M. Lewis and J.M. Haviland (eds) *Handbook of Emotions*. New York: Guilford.

Libet, B. (1993) *Neurophsiology of Consciousness*. Boston, MA: Birkhaüser.

Likert, R. (1932) A technique for the measurement of attitudes, *Archives of Psychology*, 140: 5–53.

Linn, L.S. (1965) Verbal attitudes and overt behavior: a study of racial discrimination, *Social Forces*, 43: 353–64.

Liska, A.E. (1984) A critical examination of the causal structure of the Fishbein/Ajzen attitude–behavior model, *Social Psychology Quarterly*, 47: 61–74.

Locke, K. (1996) A funny thing happened! The management of consumer emotions in service encounters, *Organizational Science*, 7: 40–59.

Loken, B. (1983) The theory of reasoned action: examination of the sufficiency assumption for a television viewing behavior, in R.P. Bagozzi and A.M. Tybout (eds) *Advances in Consumer Research*, Vol. 10. Ann Arbor, MI: Association for Consumer Research.

Loken, B. and John, D.R. (1993) Diluting brand beliefs: when do brand extensions have a negative impact?, *Journal of Marketing*, 57: 71–84.

Loken, B. and Ward, J. (1990) Alternative approaches to understanding the determinants of typicality, *Journal of Consumer Research*, 17: 111–26.

Luce, M.F. (1998) Choosing to avoid: coping with negatively emotion-laden consumer decisions, *Journal of Consumer Research*, 24: 409–33.

Lutz, K.A. and Lutz, R.J. (1977) Effects of interactive imagery on learning: application to advertising, *Journal of Applied Psychology*, 72: 493–8.

Lutz, R.J. (1975) Changing brand attitudes through modification of cognitive structure, *Journal of Consumer Research*, 1: 49–59.

Lutz, R.J. (1977) Rejoinder, *Journal of Consumer Research*, 4: 266–71.

Lutz, R.J. (1978) An experimental investigation of causal relations among cognitions, affect, and behavioral intentions, *Journal of Consumer Research*, 3: 197–208.

Lynch, J.G. (1979) Why additive utility models fail as descriptions of choice behavior, *Journal of Experimental Social Psychology*, 15: 379–417.

McArthur, L.Z. and Post, D.L. (1977) Figural emphasis and person perception, *Journal of Experimental Social Psychology*, 13: 520–35.

McGarty, C. (1999) *Categorization in Social Psychology*. London: Sage.

McGuire, W.J. (1964) Inducing resistance to persuasion: some contemporary approaches, in L. Berkowitz (ed.) *Advances in Experimental Social Psychology*, Vol. 1. New York: Academic Press.

McGuire, W.J. (1969) The nature of attitudes and attitude change, in G. Lindzey and E. Aronson (eds) *Handbook of Social Psychology*, 2nd edn, Vol. 3. Reading, MA: Addison-Wesley.

McGuire, W.J. (1985) Attitudes and attitude change, in G. Lindzey and E. Aronson (eds) *Handbook of Social Psychology*, 3rd edn, Vol. 2. New York: Random House.

McGuire, W.J. (1989) Theoretical foundations of campaigns, in R.E. Rice and C.K. Atkin (eds) *Public Communication Campaigns*, 2nd edn. Newbury Park, CA: Sage.

McGuire, W.J. and Papageorgis, D. (1961) The relative efficacy of various types of prior belief-defense in producing immunity against persuasion, *Journal of Abnormal and Social Psychology*, 62: 327–37.

MacKenzie, S.B., Lutz, R.J. and Belch, G. (1986) The role of attitude toward the ad as a mediator of advertising effectiveness: a test of competing explanations, *Journal of Marketing Research*, 23: 130–43.

Mackie, D.M. and Worth, L.T. (1989) Processing deficits and the mediation of positive affect in persuasion, *Journal of Personality and Social Psychology*, 57(1): 27–40.

Macklin, M.C. (1994) The impact of audiovisual information on children's product-related recall, *Journal of Consumer Research*, 21: 154–64.

McLaughlin, B. (1989) Type epiphenomenalism, type dualism, and the causal priority of the physical, *Philosophical Perspectives*, 3: 109–35.

Maheswaran, D. (1994) Country of origin as a stereotype: effects of consumer expertise and attribute strength on product evaluations, *Journal of Consumer Research*, 21: 354–65.

Maheswaran, D. and Chaiken, S. (1991) Promoting systematic processing in low-motivation settings: effect of incongruent information on processing and judgment, *Journal of Persuasion and Social Psychology*, 61: 13–33.

Maio, G.R., Bell, D.W. and Esses, V.M. (1996) Ambivalence and persuasion: the processing of messages about immigrant groups, *Journal of Experimental Social Psychology*, 32: 513–36.

Maison, D., Greenwald, A.G. and Bruin, R. (2001) The implicit association test as a measure of implicit consumer attitudes, *Polish Psychological Bulletin*, 32(1): 1–9.

Malle, B.F. and Knobe, J. (1997) The folk concept of intentionality, *Journal of Experimental Social Psychology*, 33: 101–21.

Mandler, G. (1982) The structure of value: accounting for taste, in M.S. Clark and S.T. Fiske (eds) *Affect and Cognition*. Hillsdale, NJ: Erlbaum.

Mano, H. and Oliver, R.L. (1993) Assessing the dimensionality and structure of the consumption experience: evaluation, feeling, and satisfaction, *Journal of Consumer Research*, 20: 451–66.

Manstead, A.S.R. and Wagner, H.L. (1981) Arousal, cognition, and emotion: an appraisal of two-factor theory, *Current Psychological Reviews*, 1: 35–54.

Marcel, A.J. (1983) Conscious and unconscious perception: an approach to the relations between phenomenal experience and perceptual processes, *Cognitive Psychology*, 15: 238–300.

Markus, H.R. and Shinobu, K. (1994) The cultural construction of self and emotion: implications for social behavior, in S. Kitayama and H.R. Markus (eds) *Emotion and Culture: Empirical Studies of Mutual Influence*. Washington, DC: American Psychological Association.

Martin, L.L., Seta, J.J. and Crelia, R.A. (1990) Assimilation and contrast as a function of people's willingness and ability to expend effort in forming an impression, *Journal of Personality and Social Psychology*, 59: 27–37.

Masson, M.E.J. (1995) A distributed memory model of semantic priming, *Journal of Experimental Psychology: Learning, Memory, and Cognition*, 21: 3–23.

Matlin, M.W. (1998) *Cognition*. Orlando, FL: Harcourt Brace.

Mazis, M.B., Ahtola, O.T. and Klippel, R.E. (1975) A comparison of four multiattribute models in the prediction of consumer attitudes, *Journal of Consumer Research*, 2: 38–52.

Medin, D.L. and Schaffer, M.M. (1978) Context theory of classification learning, *Psychological Review*, 85: 207–38.

Mele, A.R. (1992) *Springs of Action: Understanding Intentional Behavior*. Oxford: Oxford University Press.

Mele, A.R. (1995) Motivation: essentially motivation-constituting attitudes, *Philosophical Review*, 104: 387–423.

Melton, A.W. (1970) The situation with respect to the spacing of repetitions and memory, *Journal of Verbal Learning and Verbal Behavior*, 9: 596–606.

Menon, G. (1993) The effects of accessibility of information in memory on judgment of behavioral frequencies, *Journal of Consumer Research*, 20: 431–40.

Menon, G., Raghubir, P. and Schwartz, N. (1995) Behavioral frequency judgments: an accessibility-diagnosticity framework, *Journal of Consumer Research*, 22: 212–28.

Metcalfe, J. and Mischel, W. (1999) A hot/cool system analysis of delay of gratification: dynamics of willpower, *Psychological Review*, 106: 3–19.

Meyer, R.J. and Kahn, B.E. (1991) Probalistic models of consumer choice behavior, in T.S. Robertson and H.H. Kassarjian (eds) *Handbook of Consumer Behavior*. Englewood Cliffs, NJ: Prentice-Hall.

Meyers-Levy, J. (1989a) Priming effects on product judgments: a hemispheric interpretation, *Journal of Consumer Research*, 16: 76–86.

Meyers-Levy, J. (1989b) The influence of a brand name's association set size and word frequency on brand memory, *Journal of Consumer Research*, 16: 197–207.

Meyers-Levy, J. and Maheswaran, D. (1991) Exploring differences in males' and females' processing strategies, *Journal of Consumer Research*, 18: 63–70.

Meyers-Levy, J. and Peracchio, L.A. (1995) Understanding the effects of color: how the correspondence between available and required resources affects attitudes, *Journal of Consumer Research*, 22: 121–39.

Meyers-Levy, J. and Sternthal, B. (1991) Gender differences in the use of message cues and judgments, *Journal of Marketing Research*, 28: 84–96.

Meyers-Levy, J. and Tybout, A.M. (1989) Schema congruity as a basis for product evaluation, *Journal of Consumer Research*, 16: 39–54.

Meyers-Levy, J., Louie, T.A. and Curren, M.T. (1994) How does the congruity of brand names affect evaluations of brand name extensions?, *Journal of Applied Psychology*, 79: 46–53.

Mick, D.G. (1992) Levels of subjective comprehension in advertising processing and their relations to ad perceptions, attitudes, and memory, *Journal of Consumer Research*, 18: 411–24.

Mick, D.G. and Fournier, S. (1998) Paradoxes of technology: consumer cognizance, emotions, and coping strategies, *Journal of Consumer Research*, 25: 123–43.

Milberg, S.J., Park, C.W. and McCarthy, M.S. (1997) Managing negative feedback effects associated with brand extensions: the impact of alternative branding strategies, *Journal of Consumer Psychology*, 6: 119–40.

Miller, N. and Colman, D.E. (1981) Methodological issues in analyzing the cognitive mediation of persuasion, in R.E. Petty, T.M. Ostrom and T.C. Brock (eds) *Cognitive Responses in Persuasion*. Mahwah, NJ: Erlbaum.

Milliman, R.E. (1982) Using background music to affect the behavior of supermarket shoppers, *Journal of Marketing*, 46: 86–91.

Milliman, R.E. (1986) The influence of background music on the behavior of restaurant patrons, *Journal of Consumer Research*, 13: 286–9.

Miniard, P.W., Bhatla, S., Randall, L. and Rose, R.L. (1990) On the formation and relationship of ad and brand attitudes: an experimental and causal analysis, *Journal of Marketing Research*, 27: 290–303.

Mischel, W. and Patterson, C.J. (1976) Substantive and structural elements of effective plans for self-control, *Journal of Personality and Social Psychology*, 34: 942–50.

Mitchell, A.A. and Olson, J.C. (1981) Are product attribute beliefs the only mediator of advertising effects on brand attitude?, *Journal of Marketing Research*, 18: 318–32.

Mitchell, D.J., Kahn, B.E. and Knasko, S.C. (1995) There's something in the air: effects of congruent or incongruent ambient odor on consumer decision making, *Journal of Consumer Research*, 22: 229–39.

Moorman, C., Zaltman, G. and Deshpande, R. (1992) Relationships between providers and users of marketing research: the dynamics of trust within and between organizations, *Journal of Marketing Research*, 29: 314–29.

Moreau, P.C., Lehmann, D.R. and Markman, A.B. (2001a) Entrenched knowledge structures and consumer response to new products, *Journal of Marketing Research*, 38: 14–29.

Moreau, P.C., Markman, A.B. and Lehmann, D.R. (2001b) 'What is it?' Categorization flexibility and consumers' responses to really new products, *Journal of Consumer Research*, 27: 489–98.

Morrin, M. (1999) The impact of brand extensions on parent brand memory structures and retrieval processes, *Journal of Marketing Research*, 36: 517–25.

Morrin, M. and Ratneshwar, S. (2000) The impact of ambient scent on evaluation, attention, memory for familiar and unfamiliar brands, *Journal of Business Research*, 49: 157–65.

Morwitz, V.G., Greenleaf, E.A. and Johnson, E.J. (1998) Divide and prosper: consumers' reactions to partitioned prices, *Journal of Marketing Research*, 35: 453–63.

Murgraff, V., Walsh, J. and McDermott, M.R. (2000) The application of Bagozzi and Edward's theory of self-regulation to the prediction of low-risk single-occasion drinking, *Psychology, Health, and Medicine*, 5: 451–66.

Murphy, G.L. and Medin, D.L. (1985) The role of theories in conceptual coherence, *Psychological Review*, 92: 289–316.

Murray, N., Sujan, H., Hirt, E.R. and Sujan, M. (1990) The influence of mood on categorization: a cognitive flexibility interpretation, *Journal of Personality and Social Psychology*, 59(3): 411–25.

Nasby, W. and Yando, R. (1982) Selective encoding and retrieval of affectively valent information, *Journal of Personality and Social Psychology*, 43(6): 1244–53.

Nayakankuppum, D. and Priester, J.R. (2001) Attitude construction and retrieval as a function of underlying strength: a resolution of competing perspectives. Unpublished manuscript, University of Michigan.

Nisbett, R.E. and Ross, L. (1980) *Human Inference: Strategies and Shortcomings of Social Judgement*. Englewood Cliffs, NJ: Prentice-Hall.

Nisbett, R.E. and Wilson, T.D. (1977) The halo effect: evidence of unconscious alternation of judgements, *Journal of Personality and Social Psychology*, 35: 250–6.

Norman, P. and Conner, M. (1996) Predicting health-check attendance among prior attenders and non-attenders: the role of prior behavior in the theory of planned behavior, *Journal of Applied Social Psychology*, 26: 1010–26.

Norman, P. and Smith, L. (1995) The theory of planned behaviour and exercise: an investigation into the role of prior behaviour, behavioural intentions and attitude variability, *European Journal of Social Psychology*, 25: 403–15.

North, A.C., Hargreaves, D.J. and McKendrick, J. (1999) The influence of in-store music on wine selections, *Journal of Applied Psychology*, 84: 271–6.

Nowlis, S.M. and Simonson, I. (2000) Sales promotions and the choice context as competing influences on consumer decision making, *Journal of Consumer Psychology*, 9(1): 1–16.

Nyer, P.U. (1997a) A study of the relationships between cognitive appraisals and consumption emotions, *Journal of the Academy of Marketing Science*, 25(4): 296–304.

Nyer, P.U. (1997b) Modeling the cognitive antecedents of post-consumption emotions, *Journal of Consumer Satisfaction, Dissatisfaction and Complaining Behavior*, 10: 80–90.

Oatley, K. (1992) *Best Laid Schemes: The Psychology of Emotions*. Cambridge: Cambridge University Press.

Oatley, K. and Johnson-Laird, P.N. (1987) Towards a cognitive theory of emotions, *Cognition and Emotion*, 1: 29–50.

Obermiller, C. (1985) Varieties of mere exposure: the effects of processing style and repetition on affective response, *Journal of Consumer Research*, 12: 17–30.

Odedina, F.T., Hepler, C.D., Segal, R. and Miller, D. (1999) The pharmacists implementation of pharmaceutical care (PIPC) model, *Pharmaceutical Research*, 14: 135–44.

Oliver, R.L. (1980) A cognitive model of the antecedents and consequences of satisfaction decisions, *Journal of Marketing Research*, 17: 460–9.

Oliver, R.L. (1993) Cognitive, affective, and attribute bases of the satisfaction response, *Journal of Consumer Research*, 20: 418–30.

Oliver, R.L. (1994) Conceptual issues in the structural analysis of consumption emotion, satisfaction, and quality, in C.T. Allen and D.R. John (eds) *Advances in Consumer Research*, Vol. 21. Provo, UT: Association for Consumer Research.

Oliver, R.L. (1997) *Satisfaction: A Behavioral Perspective on the Consumer*. New York: McGraw-Hill.

Oliver, R.L. and Bearden, W.O. (1985) Crossover effects in the theory of reasoned action: a moderating influence attempt, *Journal of Consumer Research*, 12: 324–40.

Olney, T.J., Holbrook, M.B. and Batra, R. (1991) Consumer responses to advertising: the effects of ad content, emotions, and attitude toward the ad on viewing time, *Journal of Consumer Research*, 17: 440–53.

Olsen, G.D. (1997) The impact of interstimulus interval and background silence on recall, *Journal of Consumer Research*, 23: 295–303.

Olson, J.C. and Reynolds, T.J. (1983) Understanding consumer's cognitive structures: implications for marketing strategy, in L. Percy and A.G. Woodside (eds) *Advertising and Consumer Psychology*. Lexington, MA: Lexington Books.

Orbell, S., Hodgkins, S. and Sheeran, P. (1997) Implementation intentions and the theory of planned behavior, *Personality and Social Psychology Bulletin*, 23: 945–54.

Ortony, A., Clore, G.L. and Collins, A. (1988) *The Cognitive Structure of Emotions.* Cambridge: Cambridge University Press.

Osherson, D.N., Smith, E.E., Wilkie, O., Lopez, A. and Shafir, E. (1990) Category-based induction, *Psychological Review*, 97: 185–200.

Osgood, C.E., Suci, G.J. and Tannenbaum, P.H. (1957) *The Measurement of Meaning.* Urbana, IL: University of Illinois Press.

Ostrom, T.M. (1969) The relationship between the affective, behavioural and cognitve components of attitude, *Journal of Experimental Social Psychology*, 5: 12–30.

O'Sullivan, C.S. and Durso, F.T. (1984) Effect of schema-incongruent information on memory for sterotypical attributes, *Journal of Personality and Social Psychology*, 47: 55–70.

Ouellette, J.A. and Wood, W. (1998) Habit and intention in everyday life: the multiple processes by which past behavior predicts future behavior, *Psychological Bulletin*, 124: 54–74.

Ozanne, J.L., Brucks, M. and Grewal, D. (1992) A study of information search behavior during the categorization of new products, *Journal of Consumer Research*, 18: 452–63.

Paivio, A. (1986) *Mental Representations: A Dual Coding Approach.* New York: Oxford University Press.

Park, B. and Hastie, R. (1987) Perception of variability in category development: Istance-versus abstraction-based stereotypes, *Journal of Personality and Social Psychology*, 53 (October): 621–35.

Park, C.W., Milberg, S. and Lawson, R. (1991) Evaluation of brand extensions: the role of product feature similarity and brand concept consistency, *Journal of Consumer Research*, 18: 185–93.

Park, C.W., McCarthy, M.S. and Milberg, S.J. (1993) The effects of direct and associative brand extension strategies on consumer response to brand extensions, in L. McAlister and M.L. Rothschild (eds) *Advances in Consumer Research*, Vol. 20. Provo, UT: Association for Consumer Research.

Park, C.W., Mothersbaugh, D.L. and Feick, L. (1994) Consumer knowledge assessment, *Journal of Consumer Research*, 21: 71–82.

Park, J-W. and Hastak, M. (1994) Memory-based product judgments: effects of involvement at encoding and retrieval, *Journal of Consumer Research*, 21: 534–47.

Park, J-W. and Wyer, R.S. (1994) The cognitive organization of product information: effects of attribute category set size on information recall, *Journal of Consumer Psychology*, 2: 329–57.

Parker, D., Manstead, A.S.R. and Stradling, S.G. (1995) Extending the theory of planned behaviour: the role of personal norm, *British Journal of Social Psychology*, 34: 127–37.

Parkinson, B. (1995) *Ideas and Realities of Emotion.* London: Routledge.

Parrott, G.W. (1988) The role of cognition in emotional experience, in W.J. Baker, L.P. Mos, H.V. Rappard and H.J. Stam (eds) *Recent Trends in Theoretical Psychology.* New York: Springer-Verlag.

Peak, H. (1955) Attitude and motivation, in M.R. Jones (ed.) *Nebraska Symposium on Motivation*, Vol. 3. Lincoln, NE: University of Nebraska Press.

Pechmann, C. (1992) Predicting when two-sided ads will be more effective than one-sided ads: the role of correlational and correspondent inferences, *Journal of Marketing Research*, 29: 441–53.

Pendry, L.F. and Macrae, C.N. (1996) What the disinterested perceiver overlooks: goal-directed social categorization, *Personality and Social Psychology Bulletin*, 22: 249–56.

Peracchio, L.A. (1992) How do young children learn to be consumers: a script-processing approach, *Journal of Consumer Research*, 18: 425–40.

Peracchio, L.A. and Tybout, A.M. (1996) The moderating role of prior knowledge in schema-based product evaluation, *Journal of Consumer Research*, 23: 177–92.

Perloff, L.S. and Fetzer, B.K. (1986) Self–other judgments and perceived vulnerability to victimization, *Journal of Personality and Social Psychology*, 50: 502–10.

Perugini, M. and Bagozzi, R.P. (2001a) The role of desires and anticipated emotions in goal-directed behaviours: broadening and deepening the theory of planned behaviour, *British Journal of Social Psychology*, 40: 79–98.

Perugini, M. and Bagozzi, R.P. (2001b) The role of desires in attitude theory: conceptual issues and empirical evidence. Unpublished working paper, Essex University.

Perugini, M. and Bagozzi, R.P. (2001c) The distinction between desires and intentions. Unpublished working paper, Essex University.

Perugini, M. and Conner, M. (2000) Predicting and understanding behavioral volitions: the interplay between goals and behaviors, *European Journal of Social Psychology*, 30: 705–31.

Pervin, L.A. (1989) Goal concepts: themes, issues, and questions, in L.A. Pervin (ed.) *Goal concepts in Personality and Social Psychology*. Hillsdale, NJ: Erlbaum.

Peterson, R.E. and Thurstone, L. (1933) *Motion Pictures and the Social Attitudes of Children*. New York: Macmillan.

Peterson, R.E. and Thurstone, L. (1970) *The Effect of Motion Pictures on the Social Attitudes of High School Children*. Chicago: University of Chicago Press (original work published in 1933).

Petty, R.E. (1977) A cognitive response analysis of the temporal persistence of attitude changes induced by persuasive communications. Unpublished doctoral dissertation, Ohio State University.

Petty, R.E. (1994) Two routes to persuasion: state of the art, in G. d'Ydewalle, P. Eelen and P. Bertelson (eds) *International Perspectives on Psychological Science*, Vol. 2. Hillsdale, NJ: Erlbaum.

Petty, R.E. (1997) The evolution of theory and research in social psychology: from single to multiple effect and process models, in C. McGarty and S.A. Haslam (eds) *The Message of Social Psychology: Perspectives on Mind in Society*. Oxford: Blackwell.

Petty, R.E. and Brock, T.C. (1981) Thought disruption and persuasion: assessing the validity of attitude change experiments, in R. Petty, T. Ostrom and T. Brock (eds) *Cognitive Responses in Persuasion*. Hillsdale, NJ: Erlbaum.

Petty, R.E. and Cacioppo, J.T. (1979) Issue involvement can increase or decrease persuasion by enhancing message-relevant cognitive responses, *Journal of Personality and Social Psychology*, 37: 1915–26.

Petty, R.E. and Cacioppo, J.T. (1981) *Attitudes and Persuasion: Classic and Contemporary Approaches*. Dubuque, IA: William C. Brown.

Petty, R.E. and Cacioppo, J.T. (1984) The effects of involvement on response to argument quantity and quality: central and peripheral routes to persuasion, *Journal of Personality and Social Psychology*, 46: 69–81.

Petty, R.E. and Cacioppo, J.T. (1986) *Communication and Persuasion: Central and Peripheral Routes to Attitude Change*. New York: Springer-Verlag.

Petty, R.E. and Cacioppo, J.T. (1990) Involvement and persuasion: tradition versus integration, *Psychological Bulletin*, 107: 367–74.

Petty, R.E. and Krosnick, J.A. (eds) (1995) *Attitude Strength: Antecedents and Consequences*. Mahwah, NJ: Erlbaum.

Petty, R.E. and Wegener, D.T. (1998) Attitude change: multiple roles for persuasion variables, in D. Gilbert, S. Fiske and G. Lindzey (eds) *The Handbook of Social Psychology*, 4th edn, Vol. 1. New York: McGraw-Hill.

Petty, R.E. and Wegener, D.T. (1999) The elaboration likelihood model: current status and controversies, in S. Chaiken and Y. Trope (eds) *Dual Process Theories in Social Psychology*. New York: Guilford.

Petty, R.E., Wells, G.L. and Brock, T.C. (1976) Distraction can enhance or reduce yielding to propaganda: thought disruption versus effort justification, *Journal of Personality and Social Psychology*, 34: 874–84.

Petty, R.E., Harkins, S.G., Williams, K.D. and Latané, B. (1977) The effects of group size on cognitive effort and evaluation, *Personality and Social Psychology Bulletin*, 3: 579–82.

Petty, R.E., Harkins, S.G. and Williams, K.D. (1980) The effects of group diffusion of cognitive effort on attitudes: an information processing view, *Journal of Personality and Social Psychology*, 38: 81–92.

Petty, R.E., Cacioppo, J.T. and Goldman, R. (1981a) Personal involvement as a determinant of argument-based persuasion, *Journal of Personality and Social Psychology*, 41: 847–55.

Petty, R.E., Ostrom, T.M. and Brock, T.C. (eds) (1981b) *Cognitive Responses in Persuasion*. Mahwah, NJ: Erlbaum.

Petty, R.E., Cacioppo, J.T. and Schumann, D. (1983a) Central and peripheral routes to advertising effectiveness: the moderating role of involvement, *Journal of Consumer Research*, 10: 135–46.

Petty, R.E., Wells, G.L., Heesacker, M., Brock, T.C. and Cacioppo, J.T. (1983b) The effects of recipient posture on persuasion: a cognitive response analysis, *Personality and Social Psychology Bulletin*, 9: 209–22.

Petty, R.E., Kasmer, J.A., Haugtvedt, C.P. and Cacioppo, J.T. (1987) Source and message factors in persuasion: a reply to Stiff's critique of the Elaboration Likelihood Model, *Communication Monographs*, 54: 233–49.

Petty, R.E., Cacioppo, J.T., Sedikides, C. and Strathman, A.J. (1988) Affect and persuasion: a contemporary perspective, *American Behavioral Scientist*, 31: 355–71.

Petty, R.E., Gleicher, F. and Baker, S.M. (1991) Multiple roles for affect in persuasion, in J. Forgas (ed.) *Emotion and Social Judgments*. Oxford: Pergamon.

Petty, R.E., Cacioppo, J.T. and Haugtvedt, C. (1992) Involvement and persuasion: an appreciative look at the Sherifs' contribution to the study of self-relevance and attitude change, in D. Granberg and G. Sarup (eds) *Social Judgment and Intergroup Relations: Essays in Honor of Muzafer Sherif*. New York: Springer-Verlag.

Petty, R.E., Schumann, D.W., Richman, S.A. and Strathman, A.J. (1993a) Positive mood and persuasion: different roles for affect under high and low elaboration conditions, *Journal of Personality and Social Psychology*, 64: 5–20.

Petty, R.E., Wegener, D.T., Fabrigar, L.R., Priester, J.R. and Cacioppo, J.T. (1993b) Conceptual and methodological issues in the elaboration likelihood of persuasion: a reply to the Michigan State critics, *Communication Theory*, 3: 336–62.

Petty, R.E., Priester, J.R. and Wegener, D.T. (1994) Cognitive processes in attitude change, in R.S. Wyer and T.K. Srull (eds) *Handbook of Social Cognition*, 2nd edn, Vol. 2. Hillsdale, NJ: Erlbaum.

Petty, R.E., Haugtvedt, C.P. and Rennier, G.A. (1995a) Elaboration as a determinant of attitude accessibility. Unpublished manuscript, Ohio State University.

Petty, R.E., Haugtvedt, C.P. and Smith, S.M. (1995b) Elaboration as a determinant of attitude strength: creating attitudes that are persistent, resistant, and predictive of behavior, in R.E. Petty and J.A. Krosnick (eds) *Attitude Strength: Antecedents and Consequences*. Mahwah, NJ: Erlbaum.

Petty, R.E., Fleming, M.A. and White, P. (1999) Stigmatized sources and persuasion: prejudice as a determinant of argument scrutiny, *Journal of Personality and Social Psychology*, 76: 19–34.

Petty, R.E., Priester, J.R. and Briñol, P. (2002) Mass media and attitude change: advances in the ELM, in J. Bryant and D. Zillmann (eds) *Media Effects: Advances in Theory and Research*, 2nd edn. Hillsdale, NJ: Erlbaum.

Petty, R.E., Fleming, M.A., Priester, J.R. and Harasty Feinstein, A. (2001) Individual-versus group-interest violation: surprise as a determinant of argument scrutiny and persuasion, *Social Cognition*, 19: 418–42.

Pfau, M., Kenski, H.C., Nitz, M. and Sorenson, J. (1990) Efficacy of inoculation strategies in promoting resistance to political attack messages: application to direct mail, *Communication Monographs*, 57: 25–43.

Pham, M.T. and Johar, G.V. (1997) Contingent processes of source identification, *Journal of Consumer Research*, 24: 249–65.

Pierters, R. (1993) A control view on the behaviour of consumers: turning the triangle, *European Journal of Marketing*, 27: 17–27.

Pieters, R., Baumgartner, H. and Allen, D. (1995) A means-end chain approach to consumer goal structures, *International Journal of Research in Marketing*, 12: 227–44.

Pietroski, P.M. (2000) *Causing Actions*. Oxford: Oxford University Press.

Pittman, T.S. (1993) Control motivation and attitude change, in G. Weary, F. Gleicher and K. Marsh (eds) *Control Motivation and Social Cognition*. New York: Springer-Verlag.

Plutchik, R. (1980) *Emotion: A Psychoevolutionary Synthesis*. New York: Harper & Row.

Pratkanis, A.R., Breckler, S.J. and Greenwald, A.G. (1989) *Attitude Structure and Function*. Hillsdale, NJ: Erlbaum.

Priester, J.M. and Petty, R.E. (1996) The gradual threshold model of ambivalence: relating the positive and negative bases of attitudes to subjective ambivalence, *Journal of Personality and Social Psychology*, 71: 431–49.

Priester, J.R. and Petty, R.E. (2001) Extending the bases of subjective attitudinal ambivalence: interpersonal and intrapersonal antecedents of evaluative tension, *Journal of Personality and Social Psychology*, 80: 19–34.

Priester, J.R. and Petty, R.E. (forthcoming) The influence of spokesperson trustworthiness on message elaboration, attitude strength, and advertising effectiveness, *Journal of Consumer Psychology*.

Priester, J.R., Cacioppo, J.T. and Petty, R.E. (1996) The influence of motor processes on attitudes toward novel versus familiar semantic stimuli, *Personality and Social Psychology Bulletin*, 22: 442–7.

Priester, J.R., Wegener, D., Petty, R.E. and Fabrigar, L. (1999) Examining the psychological processes underlying the sleeper effect: the elaboration likelihood model explanation, *Media Psychology*, 1: 27–48.

Priester, J.R., Nayakankuppum, D., Fleming, M.A. and Godek, J. (2001) Evaluative processes, consideration, and choice: the influence of attitudes and attitude strength on consideration and the mediational role of consideration on the attitude to choice relationship. Unpublished manuscript, University of Michigan.

Prochaska, J.O. and Di Clemente, C.C. (1984) *The Transtheoretical Approach: Crossing Traditional Boundaries of Change*. Homewood, IL: Dorsey.

Prochaska, J.O., Di Clemente, C.C. and Norcross, J.C. (1992) In search of how people change: applications to addictive behaviors, *American Psychologist*, 47: 1102–14.

Puto, C.P. and Wells, W.D. (1984) Informational and transformational advertising: the differential effects of time, *Advances in Consumer Research*, 11: 638–43.

Raghubir, P. and Corfman, K. (1999) When do price promotions affect pretrial brand evaluations?, *Journal of Marketing Research*, 36: 211–22.

Raghubir, P. and Krishna, A. (1996) As the crow flies: bias in consumers' map-based distance judgments, *Journal of Consumer Research*, 23: 26–39.

Raghubir, P. and Krishna, A. (1999) Vital dimensions in volume perception: can the eye fool the stomach?, *Journal of Marketing Research*, 36: 313–26.

Raghubir, P. and Menon, G. (1998) AIDS and me, never the twain shall meet: the effects of information accessibility on judgments of risk and advertising effectiveness, *Journal of Consumer Research*, 25: 52–63.

Rao, A.R. and Monroe, K.B. (1989) The effect of price, brand name, and store name on buyers, *Journal of Marketing Research*, 26: 351–7.

Ratneshwar, S. and Chaiken, S. (1991) Comprehension's role in persuasion: the case of its moderating effect on the persuasive impact of source cues, *Journal of Consumer Psychology*, 18: 52–62.

Ratneshwar, S., Warlop, L., Mick, D.G. and Seeger, G. (1997) Benefit salience and consumers' selective attention to product features, *International Journal of Research in Marketing*, 14: 245–59.

Reisenzein, R. (1983) The Schachter theory of emotion: two decades later, *Psychological Bulletin*, 94: 239–64.

Reynolds, T.J. and Gutman, J. (1988) Laddering theory, method, analysis and interpretation, *Journal of Advertising Research*, 28: 11–31.

Richard, R., van der Plight, J. and de Vries, N. (1995) Anticipated affective reactions and prevention of AIDS, *British Journal of Social Psychology*, 34: 9–21.

Richins, M.L. (1997) Measuring emotions in the consumption experience, *Journal of Consumer Research*, 24: 127–46.

Roberts, J.H. and Lattin, J.M. (1997) Consideration: review of research and prospects for future insights, *Journal of Marketing Research*, 34 (August): 406–10.

Roese, N.J. and Olson, J.M. (eds) (1995) *What Might Have Been: The Social Psychology of Counterfactual Thinking*. Mahwah, NJ: Erlbaum.

Rogers, E.M. (1995) *Diffusion of Innovations*, 4th edn. New York: Free Press.

Romeo, J.B. (1991) The effect of negative information on the evaluations of brand extensions and the family brand, in R.H. Holman and R. Solomon (eds) *Advances in Consumer Research*, Vol. 18. Provo, UT: Association for Consumer Research.

Ronis, D.L., Baumgardner, M., Leippe, M., Cacioppo, J.T. and Greenwald, A.G. (1977) In search of reliable persuasion effects: I. A single session procedure for studying persistence of persuasion, *Journal of Personality and Social Psychology*, 35: 548–69.

Rosch, E.H. (1978) Principles of categorization, in E.H. Rosch and B. Lloyd (eds) *Cognition and Categorization*. Hillsdale, NJ: Erlbaum.

Rosch, E.H. and Mervis, C.B. (1975) Family resemblances: studies in the internal structure of categories, *Cognitive Psychology*, 7: 573–605.

Rose, R.L., Bearden, W.O. and Teel, J.E. (1992) An attributional analysis of resistance to group pressure regarding illicit drug and alcohol consumption, *Journal of Consumer Research*, 19: 1–13.

Roseman, I.J. (1991) Appraisal determinants of discrete emotions, *Cognition and Emotion*, 5: 161–200.

Rosenberg, M.J. (1956) Cognitive structure and attitudinal affect, *Journal of Abnormal and Social Psychology*, 53: 367–72.

Rosenberg, M.J. and Hovland, C.I. (1960) Cognitive, affective, and behavioural components of attitudes, in C.I. Hovland and M.J. Rosenberg (eds) *Attitude Organization and Change: An Analysis of Consistency among Attitude Components*. New Haven, CT: Yale University Press.

Roskos-Ewoldsen, D.R. and Fazio, R.H. (1992) The accessibility of source likeability as a determinant of persuasion, *Personality and Social Psychology Bulletin*, 18: 19–25.

Ross, B.H. and Makin, V.S. (1999) Prototype versus exemplar models in cognition, in R.J. Sternberg (ed.) *The Nature of Cognition*. Cambridge, MA: MIT Press.

Rozin, P., Haidt, J. and McCauley, C.R. (1993) Disgust, in M. Lewis and J.M. Haviland (eds) *Handbook of Emotions*. New York: Guilford.

Russell, J.A. (1980) A circumplex model of affect, *Journal of Personality and Social Psychology*, 39: 1161–78.

Russell, J.A. (1997) How shall an emotion be called, in R. Plutchick and H.R. Conte (eds) *Circumplex Models of Personality and Emotions*. Washington, DC: American Psychological Association.

Russell, J.A. and Carroll, J.M. (1999) On the bipolarity of positive and negative affect, *Psychological Bulletin*, 125: 3–30.

Russell, J.A. and Mehrabian, A. (1977) Evidence for a three-factor theory of emotions, *Journal of Research in Personality*, 11: 273–94.

Russell, J.A., Weiss, A. and Mendelsohn, G.A. (1989) Affect grid: a single-item scale of pleasure and arousal, *Journal of Personality and Social Psychology*, 57: 493–502.

Ruth, J.A., Otnes, C.C. and Brunel, F.F. (1999) Gift receipt and the reformulation of interpersonal relationships, *Journal of Consumer Research*, 25: 385–402.

Rutter, D.R. and Bunce, D.J. (1989) The theory of reasoned action of Fishbein and Ajzen: a test of Towriss's amended procedure for measuring beliefs, *British Journal of Social Psychology*, 28: 39–46.

Salovey, P. and Birnbaum, D. (1989) Influence of mood on health-related cognitions, *Journal of Personality and Social Psychology*, 57: 539–51.

Sanbonmatsu, D.M. and Kardes, F.R. (1988) The effect of physiological arousal on information processing and persuasion, *Journal of Consumer Research*, 15: 379–95.

Sanbonmatsu, D.M., Kardes, F.R. and Sansone, C. (1991) Remembering less and inferring more: effects of time of judgment on inferences about unknown attributes, *Journal of Personality and Social Psychology*, 61: 546–54.

Sanbonmatsu, D.M., Kardes, F.R. and Herr, P.M. (1992) The role of prior knowledge and missing information in multiattribute evaluation, *Journal of Organizational Behavior and Human Decision Processes*, 51: 76–91.

Schachter, S. and Singer, J.E. (1962) Cognitive, social, and physiological determinants of emotional state, *Psychological Review*, 69: 379–99.

Schaller, M. and Cialdini, R.B. (1990) Happiness, sadness, and helping: a motivational integration, in R.M. Sorrentino and E.T. Higgins (eds) *Handbook of Motivation and Cognition: Foundations of Social Behavior*, Vol. 2. New York: Guilford.

Schmitt, B.H. and Zhang, S. (1998) Language structure and categorization: a study of classifiers in consumer cognition, judgment, and choice, *Journal of Consumer Research*, 25: 108–22.

Schmitt, B.H., Tavassoli, N.T. and Millard, R.T. (1993) Memory for print ads: understanding relations among brand name, copy, and picture, *Journal of Consumer Psychology*, 2: 55–82.

Schwartz, S.H. (1992) Universals in the content and structure of values: theoretical advances and empirical tests in 20 countries, in M.P. Zanna (ed.) *Advances in Experimental Social Psychology*, Vol. 25. San Diego, CA: Academic Press.

Schwarz, N. (1990) Feelings as information: informational and motivational functions of affective states, in R.M. Sorrentino and E.T. Higgins (eds) *Handbook of Motivation and Cognition: Foundations of Social Behavior*, Vol. 2. New York: Guilford.

Schwarz, N. (1998) Accessible content and accessibility experiences: the interplay of declarative and experiential information in judgment, *Personality and Social Psychology Review: Special Issue: Metacognition*, 2(2): 87–99.

Schwarz, N. (1999) Self-reports: how the questions shape the answers, *American Psychologist*, 54(2): 93–105.

Schwarz, N. and Bless, H. (1991) Happy and mindless, but sad and smart? The impact of affective states on analytic reasoning, in J. Forgas (ed.) *Emotion and Social Judgments*. Oxford: Pergamon.

Schwarz, N. and Clore, G.L. (1983) Mood, misattribution, and judgments of well-being: informative and directive functions of affective states, *Journal of Personality and Social Psychology*, 45(3): 513–23.

Schwarz, N., Strack, F., Kommer, D. and Wagner, D. (1987) Soccer, rooms and the quality of your life: mood effects on judgments of satisfaction with life in general and with specific life domains, *European Journal of Social Psychology*, 17: 69–79.

Searle, J.R. (1983) *Intentionality: An Essay in the Philosophy of Mind*. Cambridge: Cambridge University Press.

Sen, S., Gürhan-Canli, Z. and Morwitz, V. (2001) Withholding consumption: a social dilemma perspective on consumer boycotts, *Journal of Consumer Research*, 28(3): 399–417.

Shapiro, S. (1999) When an ad's influence is beyond our conscious control: perceptual and conceptual fluency effects caused by incidental ad exposure, *Journal of Consumer Research*, 26: 16–36.

Shapiro, S., MacInnis, D.J. and Heckler, S.E. (1997) The effects of incidental ad exposure on the formation of consideration sets, *Journal of Consumer Research*, 24: 94–104.

Shaver, P., Schwartz, J., Kirson, D. and O'Connor, C. (1987) Emotion knowledge: further exploration of a prototype approach, *Journal of Personality and Social Psychology*, 52: 1061–86.

Shavitt, S., Swan, S., Lowrey, T.M. and Wänke, M. (1994) The interaction of endorser attractiveness and involvement in persuasion depends on the goal that guides message processing, *Journal of Consumer Psychology*, 3: 137–62.

Sheeran, P. and Orbell, S. (1999a) Implementing intentions and repeated behaviour: augmenting the predictive validity of the theory of planned behaviour, *European Journal of Social Psychology*, 29: 349–69.

Sheeran, P. and Orbell, S. (1999b) Augmenting the theory of planned behavior: roles for anticipated regret and descriptive norms, *Journal of Applied Social Psychology*, 29: 2107–42.

Sheppard, B.H., Hartwick, J. and Warshaw, P.R. (1988) The theory of reasoned action: a meta-analysis of past research with recommendations for modifications and future research, *Journal of Consumer Research*, 15: 325–43.

Sherif, C.W., Sherif, M. and Nebergall, R.E. (1965) *Attitude and Attitude Change: The Social Judgment-Involvement Approach*. Philadelphia, PA: W.B. Saunders.

Sherif, M. and Hovland, C.I. (1961) *Social Judgment: Assimilation and Contrast Effects in Communication and Attitude Change*. New Haven, CT: Yale University Press.

Sheth, J.N. (1972) Reply to the comments on the nature and uses of expectancy-value models in consumer research, *Journal of Marketing Research*, 9: 462–5.

Sheth, J.N. and Talarzyk, W.W. (1972) Perceived instrumentality and value importance as determinants of attitudes, *Journal of Marketing Research*, 9: 6–9.

Shimp, T.A. (1981) Attitude toward the ad as a mediator of consumer brand choice, *Journal of Advertising*, 10: 9–15.

Shimp, T.A. (1991) Neo-Pavlovian conditioning and its implications for consumer theory and research, in T.S. Robertson and H.H. Kassarjian (eds) *Handbook of Consumer Behavior*. Englewood Cliffs, NJ: Prentice-Hall.

Shimp, T.A. and Kavas, A. (1984) The theory of reasoned action applied to coupon usage, *Journal of Consumer Research*, 11: 795–809.

Shocker, A.D. and Srinivasan, V. (1979) Multiattribute approaches for product concept evaluation and generation: a critical review, *Journal of Marketing Research*, 16: 159–80.

Shrum, L.J., Wyer, R.S. and O'Guinn, T.C. (1998) The effects of television consumption on social perceptions: the use of priming procedures to investigate psychological processes, *Journal of Consumer Research*, 24: 447–58.

Simmons, C.J. and Lynch, J.G. (1991) Inference effects without inference making? Effects of missing information on discounting and use of presented information, *Journal of Consumer Research*, 17: 477–91.

Simonson, I., Huber, J. and Payne, J. (1988) The relationship between prior brand knowledge and information acquisition order, *Journal of Consumer Research*, 14: 566–78.

Smith, A. and Bolton, R. (1998) An experimental investigation of customer relations to service failure, *Journal of Service Research*, 1: 65–81.

Smith, A., Bolton, R. and Wagner, J. (1999) A model of customer satisfaction with service encounters involving failure and recovery, *Journal of Marketing Research*, 34: 356–72.

Smith, C.A. and Ellsworth, P.C. (1985) Patterns of cognitive appraisals in emotion, *Journal of Personality and Social Psychology*, 48: 813–38.

Smith, E.R. and DeCoster, J. (1999) Associative and rule-based processing: a connectionist interpretation of dual-process models, in S. Chaiken and Y. Trope (eds) *Dual-Process Theories in Social Psychology*. New York: Guilford.

Smith, E.R. and Zarate, M.A. (1990) Exemplar and prototype use in social categorization, *Social Cognition*, 8: 243–62.

Smith, E.R., Fazio, R.H. and Cejka, M.A. (1996) Accessible attitudes influence categorization of multiply categorizable objects, *Journal of Personality and Social Psychology*, 71: 888–98.

Smith, S.M. and Shaffer, D.R. (1995) Speed of speech and persuasion: evidence of multiple effects, *Personality and Social Psychology Bulletin*, 21: 1051–60.

Spangenberg, E.R., Crowley, A.E. and Henderson, P.W. (1996) Improving the store environment: do olfactory cues affect evaluations and behaviors?, *Journal of Marketing*, 60: 67–80.

Srull, T.K. (1981) Person memory: some tests of associative storage and retrieval models, *Journal of Experimental Psychology: Human Learning and Memory*, 7: 440–63.

Srull, T.K. (1983) Affect and memory: the impact of affective reactions in advertising on the representation of product information in memory, in R.P. Bagozzi and A. Tybout (eds) *Advances in Consumer Research*, Vol. 10. Ann Arbor, MI: Association for Consumer Research.

Srull, T.K. (1984) The effects of subjective affective states on memory and judgment, in T.C. Kinnear (ed.) *Advances in Consumer Research*, Vol. 11. Provo, UT: Association for Consumer Research.

Srull, T.K. and Wyer, R.S. (1979) The role of category accessibility in the interpretation of information about persons: some determinants and implications, *Journal of Personality and Social Psychology*, 37: 1660–72.

Srull, T.K. and Wyer, R.S. (1989) Person memory and judgment, *Psychological Review*, 96: 58–83.

Srull, T.K., Lichtenstein, M. and Rothbart, M. (1985) Associative storage and retrieval processes in person memory, *Journal of Experimental Psychology: Learning, Memory and Cognition*, 11: 316–45.

Staats, A.W. and Statts, C.K. (1958) Attitudes established by classical conditioning, *Journal of Abnormal and Social Psychology*, 57: 37–40.

Stangor, C., Lynch, L., Duan, C. and Glass, B. (1992) Categorization of individuals on the basis of multiple social features, *Journal of Personality and Social Psychology*, 62: 207–18.

Stayman, D.M. and Aaker, D.A. (1988) Are all the effects of ad-induced feelings mediated by Aad?, *Journal of Consumer Research*, 15: 368–73.

Stayman, D.M. and Batra, R. (1991) Encoding and retrieval of ad affect in memory, *Journal of Marketing Research*, 28: 232–9.

Stayman, D.M. and Kardes, F.R. (1992) Spontaneous inference processes in advertising: effects of need for cognition and self-monitoring on inference generation and utilization, *Journal of Consumer Psychology*, 1: 125–42.

Stayman, D.M., Alden, D.L. and Smith, K.H. (1992) Some effects of schematic processing on consumer expectations and disconfirmation judgments, *Journal of Consumer Research*, 19: 240–55.

Stein, N.L., Trabasso, T. and Liwag, M. (1993) The representation and organization of emotional experience: unfolding the emotion episode, in M. Lewis and J.M. Haviland (eds) *Handbook of Emotions*. New York: Guilford.

Stein, N.L., Liwag, M.D. and Wade, E. (1996) A goal-based approach to memory for emotional events: implementations for theories of understanding and socialization, in R.D. Kavanaugh, B. Zimmerberg and S. Fein (eds) *Emotion: Interdisciplinary Perspectives*. Mahwah, NJ: Erlbaum.

Strathman, A., Gleicher, F., Boninger, D.S. and Edwards, C.S. (1994) The consideration of future consequences: weighing immediate and distant outcomes of behavior, *Journal of Personality and Social Psychology*, 66: 742–52.

Sujan, M. (1985) Consumer knowledge: effects on evaluation strategies mediating consumer judgments, *Journal of Consumer Research*, 12: 31–46.

Sujan, M. and Bettman, J.R. (1989) The effects of brand positioning strategies on consumers' brand and category perceptions: some insights from schema research, *Journal of Marketing Research*, 26: 454–67.

Sujan, M. and Dekleva, C. (1987) Product categorization and inference making: some implications for comparative advertising, *Journal of Consumer Research*, 14: 372–8.

Sujan, M., Bettman, J.R. and Baumgartner, H. (1993) Influencing consumer judgments using autobiographical memories: a self-referencing perspective, *Journal of Marketing Research*, 30: 422–36.

Sutton, S. (1994) The past predicts the future: interpreting behaviour–behaviour relationships in social psychological models of health behaviours, in D.R. Rutler and L. Quine (eds) *Social Psychology and Health: European Perspectives*. Aldershot: Avebury.

Sutton, S. (1998) Predicting and explaining intentions and behavior: how well are we doing? *Journal of Applied Social Psychology*, 28: 1317–38.

Sutton, S., McVey, D. and Glanz, A. (1999) A comparative test on the theory of reasoned action and the theory of planned behavior in the prediction of condom use intentions in a national sample of English young people, *Health Psychology*, 18: 72–81.

Szybillo, G.J. and Jacoby, J. (1974) Intrinsic versus extrinsic cues as determinants of perceived product quality, *Journal of Applied Psychology*, 59: 74–8.

Tajfel, J. (1978) Social categorization, social identity and social comparison, in H. Tajfel (ed.) *Differentiation Between Social Groups: Studies in the Social Psychology of Intergroup Relations*. London: Academic Press.

Tajfel, J. (1981) *Human Groups and Social Categories: Studies in Social Psychology*. Cambridge: Cambridge University Press.

Tanaka, J.W. and Taylor, M. (1991) Object categories and expertise: is the basic level in the eye of the beholder?, *Cognitive Psychology*, 23: 457–82.

Tax, S. and Chandrashekaran, M. (1998) Customer evaluations of service complaint experiences: implications for relationship marketing, *Journal of Marketing*, 62: 60–76.

Taylor, S. (1994) Waiting for service: the relationship between delays and evaluations of services, *Journal of Marketing*, 58: 56–69.

Taylor, S.D., Bagozzi, R.P. and Gaither, C.A. (2001) Gender differences in the self-regulation of hypertension, *Journal of Behavioral Medicine*, 24(5): 469–87.

Teasdale, J.D. and Fogarty, S.J. (1979) Differential effects of induced mood on retrieval of pleasant and unpleasant events from episodic memory, *Journal of Abnormal Psychology*, 88(3): 248–57.

Teasdale, J.D. and Russell, L.M. (1983) Differential aspects of induced mood on the recall of positive, negative and neutral words, *British Journal of Clinical Psychology*, 22: 163–71.

Terry, D.J. and Hogg, M.A. (1996) Group norms and the attitude–behavior relationship: a role for group identification, *Personality and Social Psychology Bulletin*, 22: 776–93.

Terry, D.J., Hogg, M.A. and Duck, J.M. (1999) Group membership, social identity, and attitudes, in D. Abrams and M.A. Hogg (eds) *Social Identity and Social Cognition*. Oxford: Blackwell.

Tesser, A. (1978) Self-generated attitude change, in L. Berkowitz (ed.) *Advances in Experimental Social Psychology*, Vol. 11. New York: Academic Press.

Tetlock, P.E. (1985) Accountability: a social check on the fundamental attribution error, *Social Psychology Quarterly*, 48: 227–36.

Thurstone, L.L. (1928) Attitudes can be measured, *American Journal of Sociology*, 33: 529–54.

Towriss, J.G. (1984) A new approach to the use of expectancy value models, *Journal of the Market Research Society*, 26: 63–75.

Trafimow, D. and Sheeran, P. (1998) Some tests of the distinction between cognitive and affective beliefs, *Journal of Experimental Social Psychology*, 34: 378–97.

Tripp, C., Jensen, T.D. and Carlson, L. (1994) The effects of multiple product endorsements by celebrities on consumers' attitudes and intentions, *Journal of Consumer Research*, 20(4): 535–47.

Troutman, C.M. and Shanteau, J. (1976) Do consumers evaluate products by adding or averaging attribute information?, *Journal of Consumer Research*, 3: 101–6.

Tulving, E. (1974) Cue-dependent forgetting, *American Scientist*, 62: 74–82.

Tulving, E. and Pearlstone, Z. (1966) Availability versus accessibility of information in memory for words, *Journal of Verbal Learning and Verbal Behavior*, 5: 381–91.

Tulving, E. and Psotka, J. (1971) Retroactive inhibition in free recall: inaccessibility of information available in the memory store, *Journal of Experimental Psychology*, 87: 1–8.

Turner, J.C. (1985) Social categorization and the self-concept: a social cognitive theory of group behavior, in E.J. Lawler (ed.) *Advances in Group Processes: Theory and Research*. Greenwich, CT: JAI Press.

Tversky, A. and Kahneman, D. (1974) Judgment under uncertainty: heuristics and biases, *Science*, 185: 1124–31.

Unnava, H.R. and Burnkrant, R.E. (1991a) An imagery-processing view of the role of pictures in print advertisements, *Journal of Marketing Research*, 28: 226–31.

Unnava, H.R. and Burnkrant, R.E. (1991b) Effects of repeating varied ad executions on brand name memory, *Journal of Marketing Research*, 28: 406–16.

Unnava, H.R. and Sirdeshmukh, D. (1994) Reducing competitive ad interference, *Journal of Marketing Research*, 31: 403–11.

Urbany, J.E., Dickson, P.R. and Wilkie, W.L. (1989) Buyer uncertainty and information search, *Journal of Consumer Research*, 16: 208–14.

van den Putte, B. (1993) On the theory of reasoned action. Unpublished doctoral dissertation, University of Amsterdam.

van der Plight, J. and Eiser, J.R. (1984) Dimensional salience, judgment, and attitudes, in J.R. Eiser (ed.) *Attitudinal Judgment*. New York: Springer-Verlag.

Verbeke, W. and Bagozzi, R.P. (2000) Exploring what it means when fear rules a sales conversation, *Journal of Marketing*, 64: 88–101.

Verbeke, W. and Bagozzi, R.P. (2001a) Determinants and effects of guilt and shame by salespeople and the moderating roles of empathy and distraction cognitive style. Unpublished working paper, Erasmus University.

Verbeke, W. and Bagozzi, R.P. (2001b) The role of shame for salespeople in European and Asian cultures. Unpublished working paper, Erasmus University.

Verbeke, W. and Bagozzi, R.P. (2001c) Embarrassment and shame in salespeople and their effects on coping and performance. Unpublished working paper, Erasmus University.

Verplanken, B. and Faes, S. (1999) Good intentions, bad habits, and effects of forming implementation intentions on healthy eating, *European Journal of Social Psychology*, 29: 591–604.

Verplanken, B., Aarts, H. and van Knippenberg, A. (1997) Habit, information acquisition, and the process of making travel mode choices, *European Journal of Social Psychology*, 27: 539–60.

Verplanken, B., Aarts, H., van Knippenberg, A. and Moonen, A. (1998) Habit versus planned behaviour: a field experiment, *British Journal of Social Psychology*, 37: 111–28.

Veryzer, R.W. and Hutchinson, J.W. (1998) The influence of unity and prototypicality on aesthetic responses to new product designs, *Journal of Consumer Research*, 24: 374–94.

Viswanathan, M. and Childers, T.L. (1999) Understanding how product attributes influence product categorization: development and validation of fuzzy set-based measures of gradedness in product categories, *Journal of Marketing Research*, 36: 75–94.

Volkmann, J. (1951) Scales of judgment and their implications for social psychology, in J.H. Rohrer and M. Sherif (eds) *Social Psychology at the Crossroads*. New York: Harper.

Wansink, B. and Ray, M.R. (1996) Advertising strategies to increase usage frequency, *Journal of Marketing*, 60: 31–46.

Warner, L.G. and DeFleur, M.L. (1969) Attitude as an interactional concept: social constraint and social distance as intervening variables between attitudes and action, *American Sociological Review*, 34: 153–69.

Watson, D. and Tellegen, A. (1985) Toward a consensual structure of mood, *Psychological Bulletin*, 98: 219–35.

Watts, W.A. and Holt, L.E. (1979) Persistence of opinion change induced under conditions of forewarning and distraction, *Journal of Personality and Social Psychology*, 37: 778–89.

Weber, R. and Crocker, J. (1983) Cognitive processes in the revision of stereotypic beliefs, *Journal of Personality and Social Psychology*, 45: 961–77.

Wegener, D.T. and Petty, R.E. (1994) Mood-management across affective states: the hedonic contingency hypothesis, *Journal of Personality and Social Psychology*, 66(6): 1034–48.

Wegener, D.T., Petty, R.E. and Smith, S.M. (1995) Positive mood can increase or decrease message scrutiny: the hedonic contingency view of mood and message processing, *Journal of Personality and Social Psychology*, 69(1): 5–15.

Weiner, B. (2000) Attributional thoughts about consumer behavior, *Journal of Consumer Research*, 27: 382–7.

Westbrook, R.A. (1987) Product/consumption-based affective responses and postpurchase processes, *Journal of Marketing Research*, 24: 258–70.

Westbrook, R.A. and Oliver, R.L. (1991) The dimensionality of consumption emotion patterns and consumer satisfaction, *Journal of Consumer Research*, 18: 84–91.

Wicker, A.W. (1969) Attitudes versus actions: the relationship of verbal and overt behavioral responses to attitude objects, *Journal of Social Issues*, 25: 41–78.

Wiles, J.A. and Cornwell, T.B. (1990) A review of methods utilized in measuring affect, feelings, and emotion in advertising, *Current Issues and Research in Advertising*, 13: 241–75.

Wilkie, W.L. (1994) *Consumer Behavior*, 3rd edn. New York: Wiley.

Wilkie, W.L. and Pessemier, E.A. (1973) Issues in marketing's use of multi-attribute attitude models, *Journal of Marketing Research*, 10: 428–41.

Wittenbraker, J., Gibbs, B.L. and Kahle, L.R. (1983) Seat belt attitudes, habits, and behaviors: an adaptive amendment to the Fishbein model, *Journal of Applied Social Psychology*, 13: 406–21.

Wood, W. and Kallgren, C.A. (1988) Communicator attributes and persuasion: recipients access to attitude-relevant information in memory, *Personality and Social Psychology Bulletin*, 14: 172–82.

Wood, W., Kallgren, C.A. and Preisler, R.M. (1985) Access to attitude-relevant information in memory as a determinant of persuasion: the role of message attributes, *Journal of Experimental Social Psychology*, 21: 73–85.

Worth, L.T. and Mackie, D.M. (1987) Cognitive mediation of positive affect in persuasion, *Social Cognition*, 5: 76–94.

Yamagishi, T. and Hill, C.T. (1981) Adding versus averaging models revisited: a test of a path-analytic integration model, *Journal of Personality and Social Psychology*, 41: 13–25.

Yamagishi, T. and Hill, C.T. (1983) Initial impression versus missing information as explanations of the set-size effect, *Journal of Personality and Social Psychology*, 44: 942–51.

Yi, Y. (1989) An investigation of the structure of expectancy-value attitude and its implications, *International Journal of Research in Marketing*, 6: 71–83.

Yi, Y. (1990a) A critical review of consumer satisfaction, in V.A. Zeithaml (ed.) *Review of Marketing 1990*. Chicago: American Marketing Association.

Yi, Y. (1990b) The effects of contextual priming in print advertisements, *Journal of Consumer Research*, 17: 215–22.

Yoon, C. (1997) Age differences in consumers' processing strategies: an investigation of moderating influences, *Journal of Consumer Research*, 24: 329–42.

Zajonc, R.B. (1968) Attitudinal effects of mere exposure, *Journal of Personality and Social Psychology Monograph Supplement*, 9: 1–27.

Zajonc, R.B. (1980) Feeling and thinking: preferences need no inferences, *American Psychologist*, 35: 151–75.

Zajonc, R.B. (1984) On the primacy of affect, *American Psychologist*, 39: 117–23.

Zajonc, R.B. (1998) Emotions, in D.T. Gilbert, S.T. Fiske and G. Lindzey (eds) *The Handbook of Social Psychology*. Boston, MA: McGraw-Hill.

Zajonc, R.B. and Markus, H. (1982) Affective and cognitive factors in preferences, *Journal of Consumer Research*, 9: 123–31.

Zevon, M.A. and Tellegen, A. (1982) The structure of mood change: an idiographic/nomothetic analysis, *Journal of Personality and Social Psychology*, 43: 111–22.

Zillman, D. (1971) Excitation transfer in communication-mediated aggressive behavior, *Journal of Experimental Social Psychology*, 7: 419–34.

Zillman, D. (1983) Transfer of excitation in emotional behavior, in J.T. Cacioppo and R.E. Petty (eds) *Handbook of Social Psychology*. New York: Guilford.

Author index

Subject index

accessibility, 57, 65, 73, 141, 148–52
  see also priming
action
  definition of, 67–8
  varieties of, 68–9
  see also consumer behaviour; model of
    goal-directed behaviour; theory of
    reasoned action; theory of planned
    behaviour; theory of trying; theory
    of self-regulation
action tendencies, 38, 91
  definition of, 42
affect
  as component of attitude, 31–3
  definition of, 37–8
  measurement of, 15
  see also attitude; emotion; evaluation
affect infusion model, 63
affective commitment, 99
affective responses, 55
amygdala, 44, 53
  see also emotion
anticipated emotions, *see* emotion
appraisals
  as alternative to expectancy-value
    model, 21–2
  automatic, 92
  definition of, 39
  as part of definition of emotion, 37
  see also evaluation
appraisal theories, 39–41, 54
  see also appraisals
argument quality, 110–11

arousal, 46, 51–4
  see also emotion, definition of
assimilation and contrast, 133, 150
attention, 130–2
attitude
  accessibility, 121–2
  affective versus evaluative, 31–3
  behaviour, 124–6
  behavioural intention, 124–6
  comparison to emotions, 38, 44
  decay, 103, 122–3
  definition of, 4–5
  multidimensional models
    background, 26–7
    expectancy-value, 27–31
    global, 31–3
    goal-directed, 33–5
  one-dimensional model, 5–6
  persistence, 122–3
  resistance, 123–4
  strength, 120–7
  structure, 120–1
  toward action, 7, 13, 17, 28–30, 33,
    70, 81, 93–5
  toward ad, 55–6
  toward brand, 55
  toward failure, 4–5, 77
  toward object, 5, 7, 13–15, 17, 19–21
  toward process, 34–5, 77
  toward success, 34–5, 77
  see also anticipated emotions;
    expectancy-value model
attribution, 163–4

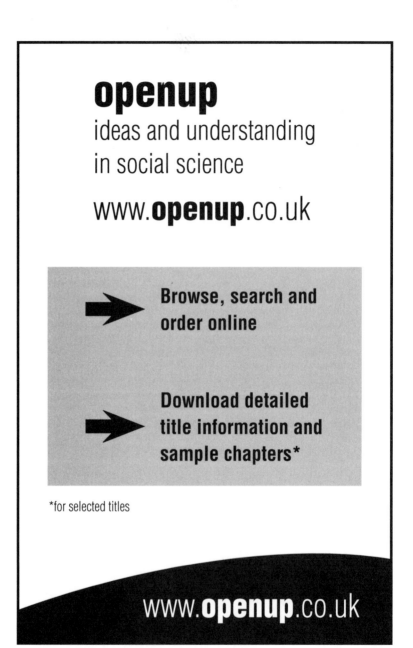